The Science of the Art of Medicine

A Guide to Medical Reasoning

John E. Brush, Jr., MD

Foreword by Harlan M. Krumholz, MD, MS

First Printing

Author:
John E. Brush, Jr., MD

Publisher:
Wayne Dementi

Graphic Designer:
Amy Mendelson Cheeley

Cover Design:
Jeffry Braun
SuperMozo Studio

Dementi Milestone Publishing, Inc.
Manakin-Sabot, VA 23103
www.dementimilestonepublishing.com

ISBN: 978-0-9909613-7-6

Dedication

Dedicated to my father, who taught me how to think.

Table of Contents

Foreword

By Harlan M. Krumholz, MD, MS

Harold H. Hines, Jr.
Professor of Medicine
and Epidemiology and
Public Health, Yale
University School of
Medicine; Co-Director,
Robert Wood Johnson
Foundation Clinical
Scholars Program, Yale
University School of
Medicine; Director, Center
for Outcomes Research
and Evaluation, Yale-New
Haven Hospital

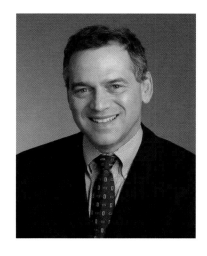

Medicine is an information science. In an earlier era, medicine moved from religion to science via laboratory work on the mechanism of disease. Doctors improved their results by reflecting on the likely cause of disease and the likely response of an individual to a treatment based on that understanding of disease. Although many benefitted from that approach, others were harmed because assumptions were not sufficiently tested empirically. There was a recognition that advances in the lab needed to be supplemented with more rigorous studies in patients, especially when the benefit was modest and not easily demonstrated. Moreover, as these studies grew, the need for doctors to be able to manage the information, understand it, and apply it wisely also grew.

Today, the expert clinician must have a command of information and know how to apply it. There is more attention than ever on the quality of treatment decisions and the assumptions that underlie them. The key to knowing how best to synthesize the available information and produce the best recommendations and decisions requires an appreciation of cognitive science.

Enter John Brush. Dr. Brush is someone who is steeped in clinical medicine, acutely aware of the daily challenges of medical decision-making, sensitive to the needs of patients, and expert in knowing where cognitive science can help. He has devoted himself to a deep understanding of the cognitive sciences, and has delivered a gem of a book that should be considered mandatory reading for all medical students and a primary reference for all practicing practitioners.

Stated simply, this book sets the foundation for clinical reasoning, providing the foundational concepts and illuminating the pitfalls that bedevil our pursuit of truth. Dr. Brush shows us why we cannot trust ourselves until we understand how we think and reason – and how we can improve our abilities by understanding the science of decision-making. He has provided a resource that is packed with wisdom and pithy chunks of knowledge that will open the eyes of many who may not have appreciated the importance of this content in medicine.

The best clinicians will always embrace the humanity of medicine - the need to connect with our patients and help them as best we can. But to be truly worthy of the trust that our patients place in us, we must invest in ensuring that we are escaping the common cognitive biases that can interfere with our best intentions to do right by them.

I have often wondered why this content does not constitute the central foundation of medical training. What is more important than the skills that enable us to navigate information, escape biases, and reach proper interpretations based on the information that is available? I have nothing against the Krebs' Cycle, but I would have been far better trained had that time been shortened and any attention at all had been paid to cognitive science. Most of our lives as clinicians are spent in the application of decision-making skills, ideally in partnership with patients, and yet so little of education in medical school and beyond is devoted to the science in this area.

Early in my training, I had the benefit of lectures by Barbara McNeil, Steven Pauker, Donald Berwick, Stephen Schoenbaum, Milton Weinstein, and Lee Goldman on the topic of decision-making. They taught me that I could best trust my own instincts if I relied on the science of decision-making. They helped me to see how often I could be mistaken if I did not realize the right way to organize information, draw from the literature, build on the science of decision-making, and fight to place the decision in the proper framework. With this book, Dr. Brush has recalled for me the excitement of realizing that it is possible to reach a greater understanding of decision-making and that such knowledge can be integrated into practice.

My best hope is that this book can stimulate a profound change in medicine. In this simple yet powerful tome, Dr. Brush has given us the capacity to change the way that practitioners think about medical decision-making and the role cognitive science can play in helping us to be better clinicians. It is time for this social science to be included in all medical core curricula and for these skills to be recognized as essential. This book is where everyone should start.

Preface

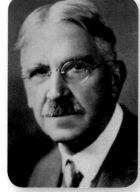

John Dewey (1859-1952)

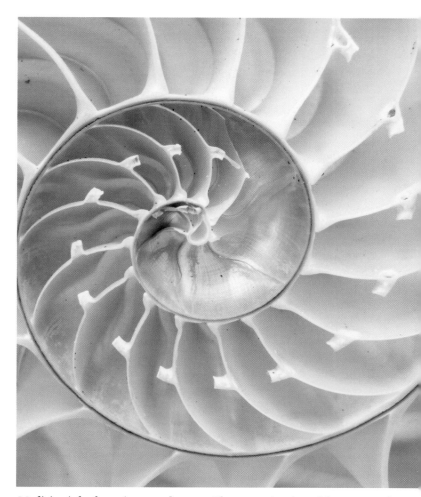

Medical education tends to focus on medical content. We teach the facts and emphasize what is known. We often assume that if we apply the facts and rules, as an engineer applies principles and equations, we can solve most medical problems. But clinical medicine is not engineering—there are simply too many missing pieces, too much uncertainty.

When faced with uncertainty, we inevitably use reasoning. But medical education gives the process of medical reasoning short shrift and rarely teaches it explicitly. We diligently teach the "what" but students often learn the "how" on their own.

Medicine is both a science and an art. Close examination of the art reveals more order and regularity than is initially apparent. Applying scientific precision and elegant simplicity can make medical care resemble a wonderful work of art.

I wrote this book to fill that gap, to aid medical students and physicians who want to improve their clinical skills through better reasoning. The book explores how sound reasoning can optimize decision making and help us avoid common pitfalls as we strive to solve medical problems.

I have become interested in medical reasoning during my three decades in medical practice. As a "reflective practitioner," to use Donald Schön's term,[2] I have aimed to improve the quality of care at my hospital and through statewide and national initiatives with the American College of Cardiology. As I worked on quality, I reflected on the thought processes that result in medical errors. My own informal "root-cause analysis" led me to the hunch that poor-quality care often stems from lapses in judgment, and Mark Graber's analysis of diagnostic error confirmed my hunch.[3] I wanted to learn more about human judgment, so I became an autodidact in the field of cognitive psychology.

I am a practicing cardiologist, so most of the examples in this book are derived from the wide array of clinical problems in cardiology. Those problems require one to draw on a variety of thinking styles, sometimes quickly and sometimes more deliberately, and cardiac problems can offer the opportunity for rapid, unequivocal feedback on clinical reasoning. Given that the field of cardiology has often led medicine in terms of clinical research and quality improvement, it provides an excellent venue for teaching medical reasoning.

This book does not present any great discoveries but, instead, synthesizes ideas that have been hiding in plain sight for years. During the past three decades, the field of cognitive psychology has developed a substantial literature on decision making but somehow hasn't had much influence on doctors, who make tough, nuanced decisions every day. I am not a cognitive psychologist, but I have learned a great deal from Herbert Simon, Gerd Gigerenzer, Daniel Kahneman, Gary Klein, and others whose work on intuition and heuristics is directly relevant to medical decision making. Influenced by the work of Ian Hacking, I have included some introductory ideas about probability, logic, and statistical inference.[4-6] I am also steeped in the literature on clinical reasoning by authors such as Alvin Feinstein, Larry Weed, Jerry Kassirer, Harold Sox, David Sackett, Pat Croskerry, Donald Redelmeier, Jerome Groopman, and Kathryn Montgomery.[7-13] I continue to learn about medical reasoning from many colleagues, too numerous to list, and I hope that this book accurately reflects their teaching.

This book follows from a series of lectures I have given to medical residents at Eastern Virginia Medical School. I developed the series when, in my practice community, I started to witness greater use of imaging and slavish adherence to oversimplified quality rules—trends that seemed to be sucking the reasoning right out of medical practice. The lecture series has been well received, and I hope that it will help our medical residents make better decisions and become better doctors. This book aims to extend that benefit to trainees in medicine outside my community.

As an introduction to the book, here is a table showing one way to classify diagnostic and therapeutic medical decisions.

Table 1. Types of medical decisions.			
	SIMPLE DECISIONS	**INTUITIVE DECISIONS**	**EVIDENCE-BASED DECISIONS**
Diagnostic	Simple recognition	Pattern recognition	Consensus-based definitions
Therapeutic	Conditional action pairs (if this, then that)	Intuitive decision making	Rules in the form of deductive syllogisms

Many decisions are simple and reactive. For instance, it's easy to recognize a broken arm or a poison ivy rash, and to prescribe a simple pain reliever. For such decisions, we use plain recognition and simple conditional action pairs, as shown in the table. Other more complex medical decisions have a well-delineated evidence base with practice guidelines to govern them, so it's just a matter of applying knowledge and working within the rules. Most of our medical decisions, however, are somewhere in between—they lack firm clinical or scientific evidence and require intuition. For example, what is the underlying cause of a patient's chest pain or shortness of breath? Should I begin treating a patient with a presumed pulmonary embolus before the diagnosis is secure?

In this book, I explain how experienced physicians use expert intuition to solve these types of medical problems.

The book begins with a reality check about the uncertainty that is an irreducible part of everyday clinical medicine. Uncertainty creates the need for reasoning, and to use it effectively we must gain an understanding of probability principles and basic cognitive psychology. Throughout the book, I show how good clinical habits can help us avoid common pitfalls that distort our judgment. I discuss specific tools, such as likelihood ratios and numbers needed to treat, which help calibrate our intuitive assessments of patients. These concepts are particularly helpful for students and trainees who are first becoming familiar with the principles of medical reasoning and how to apply them. Early learning about effective medical reasoning lays the groundwork for using it deliberately in practice in the years that follow.

In this book about intuition, I try to employ an intuitive approach in explaining concepts, using simple language and real-life examples. I also provide visual explanations to make some of the abstract ideas more accessible.

Disclaimer: I am neither a mathematician nor a philosopher, so my discussion of probability and logic may seem less than comprehensive to scholars in those fields. I simply aim to introduce the concepts sufficiently to give readers a better understanding of clinical reasoning.

Writing about how to think is a tall order. As I started this project, I reminded myself of the exhortation "physician, heal thyself." No doctor knows how to think perfectly, and I am certainly no exception. I consider myself an average thinker, certainly one less capable than our finest philosophers who have been talking and writing about thinking for millennia. Nevertheless, I hope to impart some practical wisdom that helps physicians-in-training organize their thinking. Perhaps René Descartes faced the same insecurity. In Passions of the Soul (1649), he wrote "I shall be obliged to write just as if I were considering a topic that no one had dealt with before me."

Medicine is both a science and an art. This book recognizes that there is science in the art of medicine.

References:

1. Dewey J. How we think. Boston: D.C. Heath & Co.; 1910.

2. Schön DA. The reflective practitioner: How professionals think in action. New York: Basic Books; 1983.

3. Graber ML, Franklin N, Gordon R. Diagnostic error in internal medicine. Archives of Internal Medicine. 2005; 165:1493-1499

4. Hacking I. An introduction to probability and inductive logic. Cambridge, U.K. ; New York: Cambridge University Press; 2001.

5. Hacking I. The taming of chance. Cambridge England; New York: Cambridge University Press; 1990.

6. Hacking I. Logic of statistical inference. Cambridge England, New York: Cambridge University Press; 1976.

7. Feinstein AR. Clinical epidemiology: The architecture of clinical research. Philadelphia: W.B. Saunders Co.; 1985.

8. Weed LL, Wakefield JS, Yarnall SR, Washington State Medical Record Association., Washington/Alaska Regional Medical Program. Implementing the problem-oriented medical record. Seattle: Medical Computer Services Association; 1973.

9. Kassirer JP, Wong JB, Kopelman RI. Learning clinical reasoning. Baltimore, MD: Lippincott Williams & Wilkins Health; 2010.

10. Sox HC. Medical decision making. Philadelphia: American College of Physicians; 2007.

11. Sackett DL. Clinical epidemiology: A basic science for clinical medicine. Boston: Little, Brown; 1991.

12. Groopman JE. How doctors think. Boston: Houghton Mifflin; 2007.

13. Montgomery K. How doctors think: Clinical judgment and the practice of medicine. Oxford; New York: Oxford University Press; 2006.

Chapter 1

Uncertainty in Clinical Medicine

The medical advances we have witnessed in the past half century are truly marvelous. Basic science principles are frequently and rapidly translated into practical diagnostic tests and treatments. But we are often so wowed by the progress that we lose sight of the substantial gaps in our medical knowledge.

Those gaps become readily apparent when you walk through the wards of a hospital and care directly for patients, as I do every day. Each clinical decision comes with some degree of uncertainty, and you can't discuss uncertainty without getting a bit philosophical.

Philosophers, who deal with the nature of knowledge and truth, have something to teach us about uncertainty—specifically, that it comes in two forms: epistemic and stochastic.[1,2]

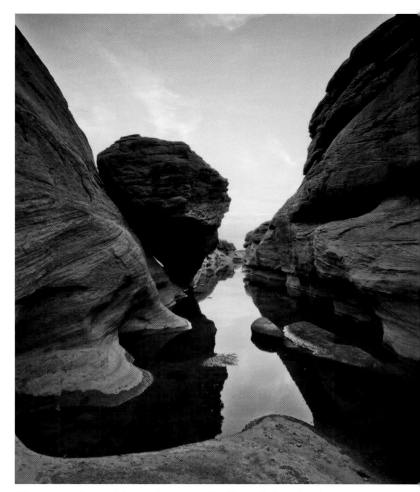

There are substantial gaps in our medical knowledge, despite enormous scientific progress and many medical advances. We bridge these gaps of uncertainty through reasoning.

Epistemic uncertainty relates to our lack of knowledge; stochastic uncertainty relates to the element of chance that affects outcomes. Epistemic uncertainty may be temporary, ultimately conquerable by medical research, but stochastic certainty (chance) will always be part of clinical medicine.

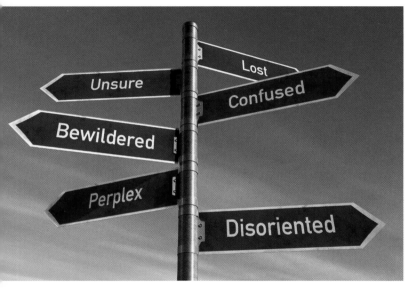

Uncertainty is a source of unease in clinical medicine. Understanding uncertainty and dealing with it directly, however, can become a source of strength.

Uncertainty in medicine can come from multiple sources, as shown in Sidebar 1.1 and enumerated below:

1. We cannot know the "true state" of a patient. Patients present with a variety of chief complaints and perplexing findings.

From the outside looking in, we find it difficult to pinpoint the problem. Patients describe their symptoms in their own words, often unclearly and illogically—and certainly not in classic textbook terms. The clinician must therefore translate the patient's history into a recognizable narrative.

Sidebar 1.1 Sources of Uncertainty in Medicine

**Epistemic Uncertainty
(Gk. episteme=knowledge)**

1. Obscure clinical findings
   The "true state" of the patient

2. Scientific ignorance
   It's unknown.
   It's known, but I don't know it.
   I don't know whether it's known or not.

3. Diagnostic, prognostic, therapeutic accuracy.

4. Complexity

**Stochastic Uncertainty
(Gk. stochastikos=to aim or to guess)**

5. Variability

6. Unpredictability

7. Likelihood of single events

Researchers tell us that expert clinicians accumulate "illness scripts" that describe prototypical presentations of various diseases.[3] To diagnose a problem, we try to match up a patient's narrative with a script stored in our memory, permitting us to reason by analogy. We become experts at linking a patient's story with our knowledge of a typical story, but an element of diagnostic uncertainty inevitably remains.

2. There is plain scientific ignorance, which we combat by becoming super-subspecialized, but not sufficiently enough to fill in every knowledge gap. Given the infinite complexity of the human body and its disease processes, perhaps infinitely more is unknown than known in medicine.

Witness the 2009 JAMA article by Tricoci and colleagues at Duke University,[4] which analyzed the strength of recommendations and evidence in 16 current cardiology guidelines. Of the 2711 recommendations in those guidelines, only 275 (10%) had an A level of evidence, meaning they were derived from multiple randomized controlled trials. Seven hundred recommendations (26%) were based on expert opinion alone, and 1736 (64%) were derived from intermediate evidence—that is, incomplete information that must be applied to practice using some degree of intuition and judgment.

What's more, this study included only written clinical practice guidelines, which capture only a portion of the problems, issues, and decisions in everyday medical care.

Therefore, relatively few clinical decisions in cardiology are based on rules and firm clinical trial evidence, and many more are based on intuition. Cognitive psychologist Gary Klein estimates that about 95% of our general everyday decisions are made by intuition,[5] not far from what the Tricoci analysis suggests regarding cardiology decisions.

3. Our diagnostic methods, predictive tools, and therapies lack perfect accuracy. For instance, stress test results are based on indirect, inherently imprecise observations. Indeed, all imaging tests have visual artifacts and measurement limitations. Even basic laboratory tests lack perfect analytic precision. Making diagnoses and predicting outcomes and treatment responses for individual patients can be fraught with inaccuracy.

4. The sheer complexity of the scientific evidence in modern medicine is daunting. No one person can possibly comprehend and retain the vast amount of medical knowledge. We are often left asking, "Is it unknown, or is it just unknown to me?"

5. Variability is mind-boggling. More than seven billion people are on the planet, and each one is unique. Even identical twins don't have identical medical problems. As individual practitioners, we see a tiny sample of that large population. By and large, the timing and circumstances of our patient encounters are chance occurrences.

6. Unpredictability is inevitable. Every patient encounter comes with a range of possibilities for the diagnosis and outcome. To enhance predictability, we use diagnostic categories, stages, and other classification schemes, but those methods are far from perfect.

7. Applying empirical evidence from populations of patients to an individual patient is very difficult. We can make highly accurate actuarial predictions for populations, but we have trouble even comprehending what probability means for a single patient or event.

Dealing with uncertainty is like groping in the dark. Darkness frightens children, and the uncertainty that is an irreducible part of clinical medicine unnerves doctors. Ironically, recognizing uncertainty and dealing with it directly can give us the confidence to go out and practice in an environment of inescapable uncertainty.

Of course, patients are sometimes attracted to doctors who create the illusion of certainty, which leads to unrealistic expectations and false hopes. An honest, open discussion about uncertainty with patients and their families is necessary to foster realistic expectations and shared decision making.

Perhaps Sir William Osler said it best: "Medicine is a science of uncertainty and an art of probability."[6] We try to counter the uncertainty with reasoning—the topic of the next chapter.

References:

1. Hacking I. The taming of chance. Cambridge England; New York: Cambridge University Press; 1990.

2. Gigerenzer G. The empire of chance: How probability changed science and everyday life. Cambridge England; New York: Cambridge University Press; 1989.

3. Bowen JL. Educational strategies to promote clinical diagnostic reasoning. N Engl J Med. 2006; 355:2217-2225

4. Tricoci P, Allen JM, Kramer JM, Califf RM, Smith SC, Jr. Scientific evidence underlying the ACC/AHA clinical practice guidelines. JAMA. 2009; 301:831-841

5. Klein, Gary. The Power of Intuition. New York: Random House; 2003.

6. Osler W, Bean RB, Bean WB. Sir William Osler aphorisms, from his bedside teachings and writings. New York: Schuman; 1950.

Chapter 2

The Logic of Medicine

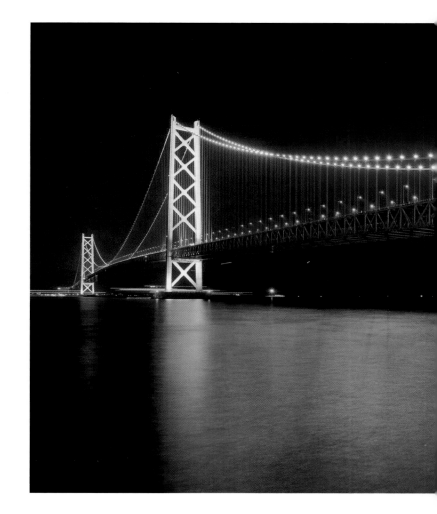

"The object of reasoning is to find out, from the consideration of what we already know, something else which we do not know."

The Fixation of Belief. Charles S. Peirce[1]

A medical diagnosis is a proposition. It can be either true or false. The field of logic gives us a framework for working with propositions. Reasoning, a mental process, uses logic to assess the truth or falsehood of propositions.

Our knowledge about logic comes from many thinkers over centuries, starting with Greek philosophers, like Aristotle, in the fourth century B.C.[1] In medicine, we didn't invent our own rules of logic — we borrowed them from longstanding general principles. Let's touch on them briefly.

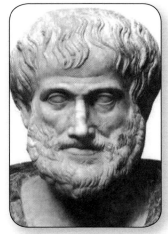

Aristotle (384 BC-322 BC)

Logic is about arguments. In logic, an argument is not a quarrel but a set of reasons that lead to a conclusion. An argument is sound if the reasons are true and the logic is valid.

Consider this logical argument: Patients with myocardial infarction derive a survival benefit from treatment with beta-blockers. My patient has a myocardial infarction. Therefore, my patient will derive a survival benefit from beta-blocker therapy. That is a sound argument.

Logical arguments consist of propositions. These statements are either premises or conclusions, and they are true or false. A valid argument that is based on true premises is a sound argument.

There are two principal forms of arguments and reasoning: deductive and inductive (Figure 2.1). A deductive argument consists of premises that state a general principle and lead to a conclusion about a particular case. With deductive reasoning, the truth of the premises guarantees the truth of the conclusion. A scientific argument that can be made into the form of a deductive argument makes a very strong case because that type of argument is considered watertight. Deductive arguments are risk-free.

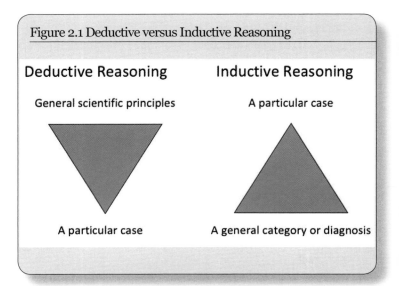

Figure 2.1 Deductive versus Inductive Reasoning

Deductive Reasoning

General scientific principles

A particular case

Inductive Reasoning

A particular case

A general category or diagnosis

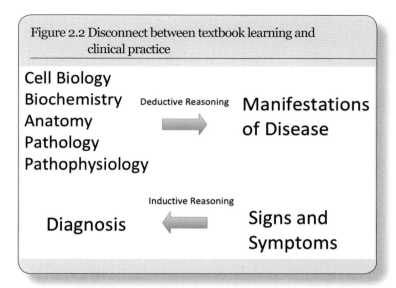

Figure 2.2 Disconnect between textbook learning and clinical practice

Aristotle taught us about deductive reasoning and its common fallacies (errors). Philosophical discussions, dating back to Aristotle and continuing for many centuries, have indirectly influenced the development of medical reasoning.

The scientific principles and rules we learn in textbooks often take the form of deductive arguments (syllogisms). In the basic sciences, general principles help us reach conclusions about particular patients (Figure 2.2). Clinical rules also take the form of deductive arguments, as in the aforementioned example about beta-blocker use after acute myocardial infarction.

Inductive Reasoning

Most dilemmas in clinical medicine don't lend themselves to deductive reasoning. We start with a premise about a particular patient and attempt to make a generalization about that patient using inductive reasoning. With inductive reasoning, the truth of the premises doesn't guarantee the truth of the conclusion. Inductive reasoning involves a degree of probability, making inductive arguments inherently risky. Consider this inductive argument:

Premise 1: My patient with chest pain has a positive troponin test.

Premise 2: A troponin test is positive in patients with myocardial infarction.

Conclusion: My patient is probably having a myocardial infarction.

The inductive conclusion is not guaranteed to be true. It is inherently risky because, unlike in a deductive argument, it involves a degree of probability and is not watertight. Therefore, to use inductive reasoning, we must understand probability.

David Hume, one of the most influential philosophers who ever wrote in English, discussed "the problem of induction" in his seminal work *An Enquiry Concerning Human Understanding*. He was skeptical about induction because logic could not guarantee the truth of the conclusion. He was concerned that inductive, probabilistic arguments assume that the future will repeat the past. Nevertheless, he said that inductive reasoning is necessary for many everyday decisions in life:

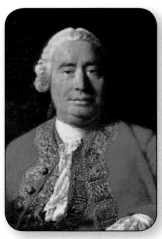

"It is not, therefore, reason, which is the guide to life, but custom. That alone determines the mind in all instances to suppose the future conformable to the past. However easy this step may seem, reason would never, to all eternity, be able to make it."[2]

Just as Hume stated hundreds of years ago, it is still often custom and habit, not reason, that guide us in daily clinical practice.

The Scottish philosopher, David Hume (1711-1776)

Some years after Hume, the Reverend Thomas Bayes formulated a rational way to reason from experience, creating an evasion of Hume's problem of induction. To deal with the inverse logic of inductive reasoning, Bayes invented a way to calculate inverse probability. (We will return to the Reverend Bayes in Chapter 3).

Forcing ourselves to use deductive instead of inductive reasoning can sometimes lead to logical fallacies, such as this one: "If a patient has a myocardial infarction, then the

---

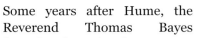

Inductive Reasoning

Truth of premises doesn't guarantee the truth of the conclusion. It involves a degree of probability.

PREMISE:
My patient with chest pain has a positive troponin.

The troponin is positive in patients with MI.

CONCLUSION:
My patient is having an MI.

Well... not necessarily.

My patient is probably having an MI.

troponin test is positive. My patient's troponin test is positive. Therefore, my patient has a myocardial infarction."

We see this logical fallacy in emergency rooms and hospitals every day. Consider this similar scenario: "If James wants a job, then he will get a haircut. James got a haircut. Therefore, James wants a job." This example (borrowed from Ian Hacking[1]) makes the mistake more obvious. James might get a haircut for a variety of reasons. Maybe his mother is coming to visit. Maybe he has a regularly scheduled haircut. Similarly, there are other reasons for a positive troponin test. The patient may have renal failure, for instance, or pericarditis. It would be a mistake to infer that a positive troponin test is conclusive evidence for a myocardial infarction.

This is a fallacy that Aristotle called "affirming the consequent." When the first premise of a logical argument is an if-then statement, the "if" portion is the antecedent (if a patient has a myocardial infarction; if James wants a job) and the "then" statement is the consequent (then the troponin is positive; then he will get a haircut). When the second premise simply affirms the consequent, a logical error occurs. We can frame the rules of medicine as deductive arguments, but when we use deductive arguments incorrectly, we can make mistakes. In situations that involve uncertainty and probability, deductive reasoning doesn't work. Rather than trying to force a deductive argument, resulting in a fallacy, we have to rely on a different type of argument. In situations when we try to draw a general conclusion about a particular case, we use inductive reasoning.

Abductive Reasoning

One other type of reasoning bears mentioning. "Abductive reasoning," described by pragmatic philosopher Charles Sanders Peirce,[3] is reasoning toward a plausible hypothesis to infer the best explanation. Science abounds with such examples, such as the big bang theory. We cannot know the final answer, or the probability of a theory, so we reason toward the most plausible hypothesis.

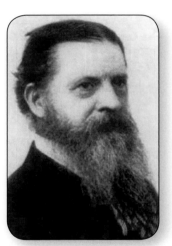

Charles Sanders Peirce (1839-1914)

Consider this poignant example of abductive reasoning: You learn that a patient of yours, Mr. Smith, died suddenly. He was a 70-year-old man whom you had treated for hypertension and hyperlipidemia for many years. A stress test a year ago was negative. Unfortunately, Smith continued to smoke. He collapsed at home. The emergency medical technicians found him to be in ventricular fibrillation, and he could not be resuscitated. An autopsy was not performed.

We use abductive reasoning to create a hypothesis about the cause of Mr. Smith's death. Abductive reasoning, according to Peirce, is neither inductive nor deductive reasoning, but could be considered a blend of both. Inductive reasoning tells us that the cause of Mr. Smith's death likely was an acute myocardial infarction. Deductive causal reasoning supports the hypothesis, given what is known about how atherosclerotic plaque rupture can lead to myocardial necrosis and lethal ventricular arrhythmias. The example shows how we use abductive reasoning to form a hypothesis that, if true, would explain the puzzling phenomenon.

Kathryn Montgomery, a humanities scholar at Northwestern University, has observed doctors in practice for many years. In her book *How Doctors Think*,[4] she states that doctors frequently use abductive reasoning in clinical medicine. Take the everyday example of a patient with new systolic heart failure and hypertension. In such cases, we often don't learn the underlying cause of the patient's dilated cardiomyopathy. Using abductive reasoning, we may decide that the most likely cause is longstanding hypertension. Other diagnoses are considered, and correctable causes are ruled out. We decide that hypertension is the most plausible hypothesis, but we may never know for sure.

Montgomery also asserts that doctors use "thinking in action," which Aristotle called "phronesis." MIT social scientist Donald Schön wrote about this type of thinking in his book *The Reflective Practitioner*.[5] He described how many types of professionals, including doctors and engineers, use learned habits and creative improvisation to solve problems. They have to rely on risky arguments or reason toward a plausible hypothesis, rather than absolutely conclusive deductive arguments. The nature of their business requires inductive and abductive reasoning.

Intuitive vs. Analytical Modes of Thinking

Discussing the logic of medicine implies that people can, and are willing to, use deliberative logic to solve problems. However, cognitive psychologists like Princeton's Daniel Kahneman note that we are not always purely rational in making decisions.[6] We constantly seek to ease cognitive strain and sometimes use shortcuts. Psychologists describe the modularity in our thinking as two essential modes: intuitive (System 1 thinking) and analytical (System 2 thinking).

To understand System 1 thinking and its potential mistakes, consider this word problem: "A bat and a ball cost $1.10 in total. The bat costs $1.00 more than the ball. How much does the ball cost?"

System 1 thinking wants you to blurt out 10¢. Fortunately, System 2 thinking checks your answer and yields the correct answer: 5¢. System 1 tries to substitute an easier question: Rather than "the bat costs $1.00 more than the ball," which requires some calculating, it substitutes "the bat costs $1.00," which requires no calculating. This quick-and-dirty shortcut, prompted by the way the question is framed, leads System 1 to make the mistake.

Here is an alternative framing: "A bat and a ball cost $1.10 total. The bat costs $1.05. How much does the ball cost?" This framing offers no invitation to oversimplify and make a mistake. A simple, more direct question can set up System 1 to succeed rather than fall into a trap.

Consider these contrasts between System 1 and System 2: System 1 thinking is fast, automatic, and intuitive; System 2 thinking is slow, deliberate, and analytical.

System 1 looks for quick, easy answers; System 2 is consciously effortful and plodding.

System 1 thinking is like driving a car on a highway, almost mindless; System 2 is like parking a car in a tight space, cautious and meticulous.

System 1 uses association and metaphor, and it loves stories; System 2 uses explicit language and beliefs, and it makes reasoned choices.

System 1 sees the forest; System 2 sees the trees.

The bat-and-ball example shows how System 1 often substitutes an easy question for a hard one, which can set up a trap. System 1 can lead to fallacies, biases, and illusions. Yet System 1 thinking is often right.

System 1 Thinking

1. Fast, automatic, intuitive.

2. Looks for quick, easy answers.

3. Driving.

4. Uses association, metaphor, loves stories.

5. Sees the forest.
   - Substitutes an easy question for a hard question.
   - Fallacies, biases, illusions.
   - Often right.

System 2 Thinking

1. Slow, deliberate, analytical.

2. Consciously effortful, plodding.

3. Parking in a tight space.

4. Explicit beliefs and reasoned choices.

5. Sees the trees.
   - Why not always use System 2 thinking in medicine?
   - Too slow.
   - Can't handle uncertainty.

So why not always use our analytical System 2 thinking in medicine? Simply because it's too slow and can't handle uncertainty. System 1 thinking uses heuristics (mental shortcuts) to make rapid decisions when the full facts are unknown. To make rapid decisions in suboptimal conditions, we "satisfice," a concept from Herbert Simon[7] that we'll discuss in chapter 5.

To overcome some of the deficiencies, we can tame our System 1 thinking. Learned habits, such as a standardized history and physical or formulating a differential diagnosis, are ways we can tame our System 1 impulses and avoid jumping to conclusions. Metacognition, an executive function that we use to monitor our thinking, allows us to double-check System 1. When System 1 thinking fails, it is usually because it moved too fast, misunderstood the question, or failed to account for all the variables. System 2's double-checking can help avoid the common pitfalls.

Because of uncertainty, medical reasoning requires the use of System 1's intuition. Psychologists tell us that skilled intuition enables three functions: classifying, estimating, and choosing. Interestingly enough, those intuitive tasks can answer the three questions that, according to Dr. Jordan Cohen, all patients ask their doctor: What is happening to me? What is going to happen to me? What can you do for me?[8] We use skilled intuition to estimate our answers to the three questions, and the answers are medical care's deliverables: a diagnosis, a prognostic estimate, and a treatment plan.

PATIENT'S QUESTIONS	SKILLED INTUITION	MEDICAL PROCESSES
Doc, what is happening to me?	Classify	Diagnosis
Doc, what is going to happen to me?	Estimate	Prognosis
Doc, what can you do for me?	Choose	Treatment

Medical reasoning requires that we use intuition and inductive reasoning. Inductive reasoning relies on risky, probabilistic arguments. Probability is the subject of our next chapter.

References:
1. Hacking I. An introduction to probability and inductive logic. Cambridge, U.K. ; New York: Cambridge University Press; 2001.

2. Hume D, Selby-Bigge LA (editor). An Enquiry Concerning Human Understanding. Reprinted from the posthumous edition of 1777 and edited by L.A.Selby-Bigge, University College, Oxford. Second Edition (on Amazon Kindle Edition); 1902.

3. Peirce CS, Houser N, Kloesel CJW, Peirce Edition Project. The essential Peirce : Selected philosophical writings. Bloomington: Indiana University Press; 1992.

4. Montgomery K. How doctors think: Clinical judgment and the practice of medicine. Oxford; New York: Oxford University Press; 2006.

5. Schön DA. The reflective practitioner: How professionals think in action. New York: Basic Books; 1983.

6. Kahneman D. Thinking, fast and slow. New York: Farrar, Straus and Giroux; 2011.

7. Simon, H. A. (1956). "Rational choice and the structure of the environment." Psychological Review, Vol. 63 No. 2, 129-138.

8. Cohen, JJ. Remembering the Real Questions. Ann Intern Med 1998: 129(7);563-6.

Chapter 3

Probability: Uncertainty Quantified

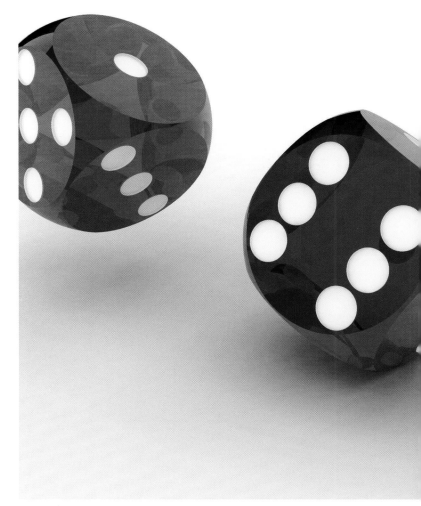

An old adage holds that nothing in medicine is either zero or one hundred percent. In other words, certainties are very rare. When chances are neither zero nor one hundred percent, what are they? Probability helps us quantify the chances that an event will occur or that a proposition will turn out to be true. It allows us to estimate the chances that a procedure will be uncomplicated or that a diagnosis will be accurate. Probability enables us to make calculated bets and educated guesses. Good use of probability leads to better judgments, resulting in better outcomes. A good understanding of probability is key to inductive reasoning. The ability to accurately estimate probability is the hallmark of a good physician.

Probability gives us a way to explain variation. Patients come in all shapes and sizes. A large group of patients will have a range of possible weights, heights, blood glucose levels—you name it. If you piled up the data on a group of patients, most of it would accumulate in the middle of the range and some would scatter to the edges, like grains of sand (Figure 3.1).

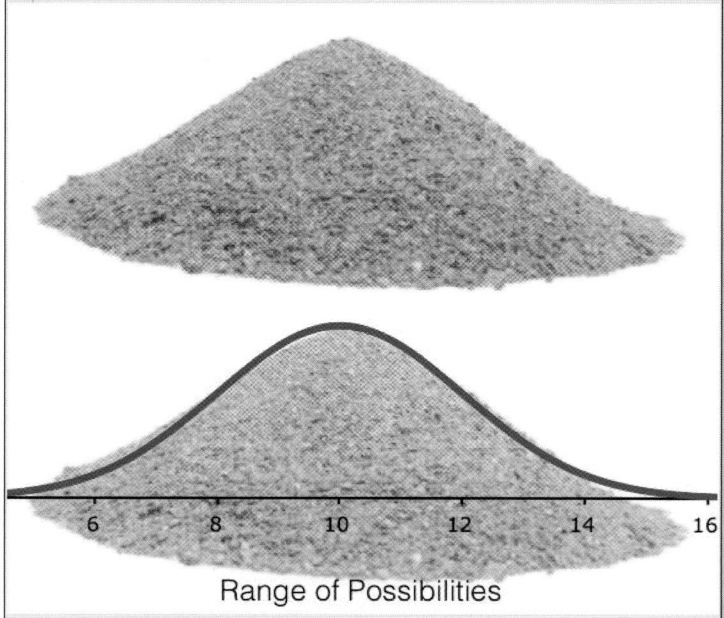

Consider the body weight of patients treated in an emergency room. Most patients would cluster in the middle of the range; fewer would scatter to the edges of the range of possible weights. For a continuous variable like weight, we can use a probability density curve to graph how patients are distributed, as shown in Figure 3.2.

Figure 3.1 Probability density is similar to a pile of sand, where most of the grains accumulate in the middle and some scatter to the edges.

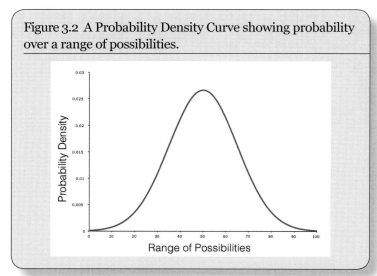

Figure 3.2 A Probability Density Curve showing probability over a range of possibilities.

It is amazing how much of nature and medicine can be described by a normal distribution, or a bell-shaped curve. For populations whose data aren't naturally distributed as a bell-shaped curve, the distribution can be easily transformed into a bell-shaped curve by taking repeated samples of the population. Central limit theorem tells us that for any population distribution, if you take repeated samples, the sample means will assume a normal distribution. Taking more samples and increasing the sample size make the distribution of the sample means look increasingly like a perfect bell-shaped curve. Interestingly, the mean of the transformed bell-shaped distribution will be the same as the mean of the original distribution.

A probability density curve (Figure 3.3) can be defined by an index of central tendency—such as the mean (the average), the median (the halfway point between the upper and lower half of the distribution), or the mode (the point that has the

highest probability density)—and an index of dispersion, usually the standard deviation. The curve may be symmetric, as shown, or it may be asymmetric (skewed).

Cumulative probability is the sum of the probabilities within a set range of possibilities. A cumulative probability curve (Figure 3.4, in red) shows how all the probabilities across the entire range of possibilities add up to one. Moving from left to right across the continuum of possibilities on the x-axis, any point on the cumulative probability curve equals the sum of the probabilities of all the possibilities to the left of the

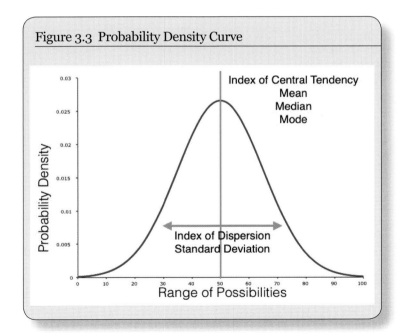

Figure 3.3 Probability Density Curve

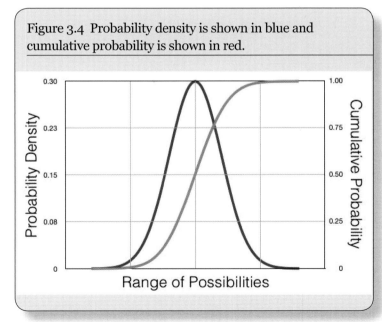

Figure 3.4 Probability density is shown in blue and cumulative probability is shown in red.

corresponding point on the x-axis. Imagine an ant walking over the pile of sand in Figure 3.1. The cumulative probability would be similar to the total amount of sand that the ant had crossed at each point as it walked from left to right over the pile. Appendix 1 includes more information about probability curves.

A probability distribution is shown in Figure 3.5. Here the probabilities of several discrete independent possibilities are shown. I have chosen to display the categorical possibilities in an order that resembles a bell-shaped curve, but for nominal

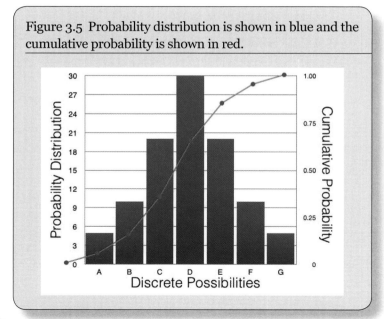

Figure 3.5 Probability distribution is shown in blue and the cumulative probability is shown in red.

variables, the possibilities could be displayed in any order. Again the cumulative probability curve, shown in red, reveals how the probabilities of all the possibilities add up to one. Having a mental picture of these ideas will help us understand how to apply probability in practice.

The Meaning of Probability

Understanding the meaning of probability is not easy. Philosophers and mathematicians have been arguing about it for centuries. For the most part, our understanding of probability developed outside the realm of medicine. Most doctors don't learn about how probability ideas developed and don't stop to think about what probability really means. Philosopher of science Ian Hacking has written several very interesting books about probability.[1-3] He notes that people have been throwing dice and casting lots for much of recorded history, but they did not begin to use mathematical calculations of probability until around 1650–1700. The world was entering the age of enlightenment and an age of reason. Authoritarian dictates of monarchs and clergy were being questioned. People began to recognize the value of an individual's ability to reason. People's long-held belief in determinism was replaced by a realization that there is some randomness to life. Thinkers like Blaise Pascal started to think about quantifying predictions.

About this time, there was an abundance of data that could be analyzed, leading to the emergence of financial products like annuities and life insurance. The emergence of these financial products created a need to calculate probability.

Some of the key people who helped develop the meaning of probability are listed in Sidebar 3.1. Scanning this history reveals several interesting points. One is that mathematical calculation of probability developed so late in history. The Greek philosophers had a lot to say about logical thinking, but it wasn't until thousands of years later that people developed a mathematical understanding of probability.

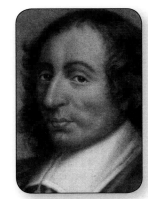

Blaise Pascal (1632-62) developed the first ideas about quantifying probability and using probability calculations to improve outcomes.

Interestingly, ideas about probability developed independently of the field of medicine. Doctors didn't think formally about probability until the 1920s, when statistics became a discipline in its own right. And it was the push for "evidence-based medicine" — a relatively recent event — that prompted practicing physicians to quantify probability (as a

Sidebar 3.1 The Development of Probability Ideas

Blaise Pascal (1623-62) Letter to Pierre de Fermat about dividing stakes of an interrupted game. Pascal's Wager and Decision Analysis.

Christian Huygens (1629-95) Expected value.
In 1657 he wrote *De Aleae*.

Jacques Bernoulli (1654-1705) Law of Large Numbers.

Abraham de Moive (1667-1754) *The Doctrine of Chances*.

Wilhelm Leibniz (1646-1716) Degrees of proof in law.

Pierre Laplace (1749-1827) First text on probability.

Thomas Bayes (1702-61) Bayes Rule.

David Hume (1711-76) The induction problem.

C. F. Gauss (1777-1855) Studied probability curves.

John Venn (1824-1923) English logician, Venn diagrams.

Charles S. Peirce (1839-1914) Abductive reasoning.

Karl Pearson (1857-1936) Correlation, Chi-squared test.

R. A. Fisher (1890-1962) Significance testing. Randomized Controlled Trials.

Jerzy Neyman (1894-1981) E.S.Pearson (1895-1980) Statistical hypothesis testing, statistical power.

Bruno de Finetti (1906-1985) Personal probability.

A. N. Kolmogorov (1903-1987) Definitive axioms for probability theory.

John Maynard Keynes (1883-1946)
Treatise on Probability. Personal probability.

number) when deciding how to care for individual patients. Two distinct notions of probability eventually took shape:

• The frequentist notion, endorsed by people like R.A. Fisher, views probability as a distribution of measurements or observations (Figure 3.6). The idea is that probability derives objectively from empirical data and physical outcomes. The frequentist notion looks backward: It measures past events and describes what happens over the long run. It uses an index of central tendency (usually the mean of the measured observations) and an index of dispersion of the observations (usually the standard deviation).

• The personal notion, endorsed by people like Bruno de Finetti, views probability as a question of future likelihood. Also called Bayesian probability (after The Rev. Thomas Bayes), the personal notion looks forward: The index of central tendency is not the mean, but an estimate of likelihood; the central point estimate is your degree of belief or conviction about a proposition or the chances of an occurrence (Figure 3.7). The dispersion is a second-order probability, or the degree of ambiguity around that belief

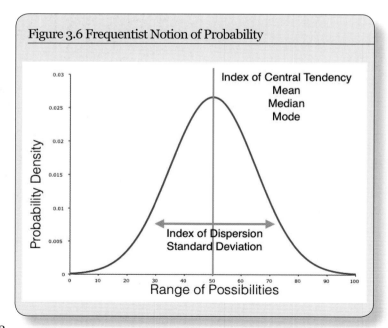

Figure 3.6 Frequentist Notion of Probability

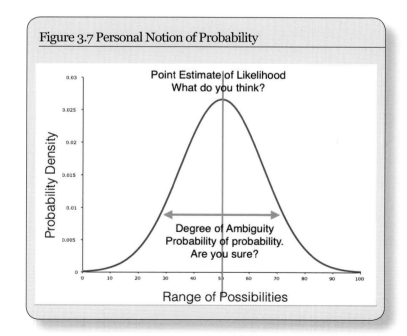

Figure 3.7 Personal Notion of Probability

or conviction. Bayesians ask, "What do I think?" and "Am I sure?"

One personal probability dogmatist was John Maynard Keynes, the economist famous for his theory of supply side economics. Keynes was also a brilliant mathematician who wrote *Treatise on Probability*.[3] Keynes scoffed at the frequentists, who viewed probability over the long run, by famously saying, "Over the long run, we will all be dead."

These dual notions of probability enable us to apply observational data to individual patients. When we inform a patient about probability, we shift from a frequentist to a personal point of view. As a frequentist, we can calculate operative mortality rates for a procedure by looking back at data from a registry, a clinical trial, or our own aggregated experience. To explain the probability of a future event to an individual patient, however, we have to shift to a personal probability point of view. If we tell a patient that his operative mortality rate is 10%, he may ask, "What do you mean doc? For me, the mortality is either 0 or 100%?" What you really mean is that you are 90% sure that the patient will survive the operation. Physicians learn with experience to flip back and forth from one notion of probability to the other, depending on the circumstances.

This personal notion of probability is the essence of inductive reasoning. However, the philosopher David Hume pointed out many years ago that the validity of this form of reasoning depends on the assumption that past observations will repeat themselves in the future.

Mental Models of Probability

Many mental models can help us think about probability and chance setups. There is the toss of a fair coin, rolling dice, drawing a random card from a deck, buying a lottery ticket, and drawing balls from an urn. There are bets, odds on bets, and point spreads. To help quantify probability, it is sometimes helpful to compare the chances of a proposition or prediction to the odds of a bet or the fair price of a lottery ticket. This can help put a number on one's conviction or degree of belief about a particular outcome. A similar exercise is the standard

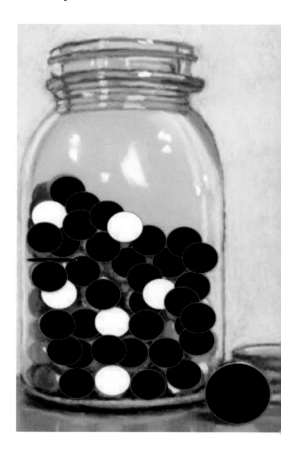

A variety of models, such as drawing balls from an urn, help us visualize the idea of probability.

reference gamble, a technique to determine whether a person would be willing to make a particular choice, compared with another choice with known probabilities and consequences. All of these models can help us grasp the quantitative meaning of probability and chance.

Simple, Compound, and Conditional Probability

Probability can be simple, compound, or conditional. A simple probability could be the chance of getting heads when tossing a fair coin, the chance of getting a one when throwing a die, the chance of getting struck by lightning, or the chance of being on call the night a random patient came to the emergency room with a heart attack and cardiogenic shock.

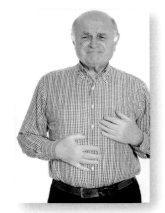

Patient with sharp chest pain of several months duration.

Compound and conditional probabilities require more thought and calculation than a simple probability. To understand compound probability, consider this example: A patient comes to your office complaining of sharp intermittent chest pain that has persisted for several months. You may start to think about a range of possible diagnoses. He clearly has something wrong with him, and there doesn't seem to be a reason to suspect multiple diagnoses.

Figure 3.8 shows a range of possible diagnoses and provisional baseline probabilities, which we might assign based on our own experience. If the possible diagnoses are mutually exclusive (no overlap) and they are collectively exhaustive (it has to be one of them), then the sum of the probabilities of all the possibilities will add up to 1 (or 100%). The range of possibilities, called the sample space, may vary depending on whether the patient is seen in an emergency room, a primary care office, or a cardiologist's office. We might group patients with chest pain into different sample spaces depending on their age, gender, type of pain, and cardiovascular risk factors. Using these patient characteristics, we can group patients into diagnostic categories with different baseline probabilities.

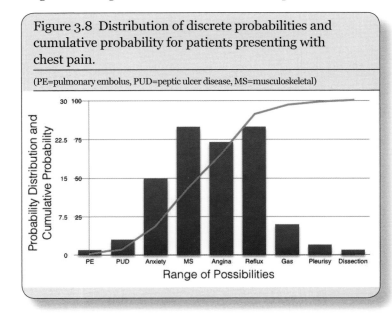

Figure 3.8 Distribution of discrete probabilities and cumulative probability for patients presenting with chest pain.

(PE=pulmonary embolus, PUD=peptic ulcer disease, MS=musculoskeletal)

For example, we would assign a lower baseline probability of angina to a young woman with no risk factors and atypical chest pain than to an elderly man who smokes and has exertional chest tightness. As suggested by the error bars in Figure 3.9, ambiguity surrounds our estimates of probability for each possible diagnosis. As we take additional history, perform a physical examination, and collect more data, the probability of the various diagnostic possibilities may rise or fall and the ambiguity may diminish as we begin to converge on the most likely diagnosis (Figure 3.10). To make a diagnosis, we make mental calculations to estimate the relative probabilities of all the possible diagnoses.

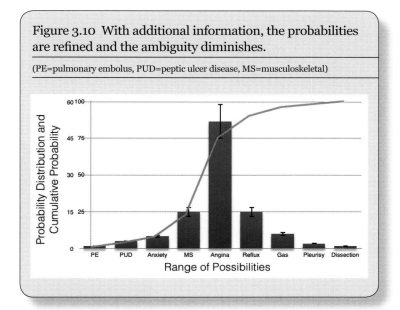

Figure 3.10 With additional information, the probabilities are refined and the ambiguity diminishes.

(PE=pulmonary embolus, PUD=peptic ulcer disease, MS=musculoskeletal)

To calculate the probability of multiple events or propositions, we need to review some probability principles:

1. The probability of an event or proposition (like a diagnosis) is: $0 < p(A) < 1$, where 0 = an impossibility and 1 = a certain event.
2. Probabilities of independent events that are mutually exclusive (no overlap) and collectively exhaustive (it has to be one of them) add up to 1.
3. The compound probability for either of 2 independent and mutually exclusive events occurring can be expressed as: $p(A \text{ or } B) = p(A) + p(B)$.

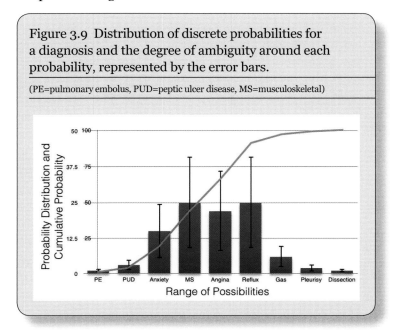

Figure 3.9 Distribution of discrete probabilities for a diagnosis and the degree of ambiguity around each probability, represented by the error bars.

(PE=pulmonary embolus, PUD=peptic ulcer disease, MS=musculoskeletal)

4. The compound probability for two independent events both occurring can be expressed as:
p(A and B) = p(A) x p(B).

The latter equation shows that two independent events both occurring is less likely than either one occurring by itself. This equation provides a justification for the law of parsimony, or Occam's Razor (attributed to William of Ockham, who proposed that the simplest solution is always the best one). Most likely, clinical findings will be due to a single diagnosis, rather than multiple diagnoses, simply because the probability of two independent events occurring simultaneously is the product of each individual probability. Each probability is a fraction, so the product of multiple probabilities will be less than each probability by itself.

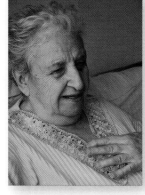
A patient comes to the emergency room with chest pain. The troponin is slightly elevated.

Conditional probability is the probability that something will happen, on the condition that something else happens. In clinical medicine, we use conditional probabilities almost constantly. Consider the following example: A patient comes into the emergency room with chest pain. The pain is now gone. The EKG is normal, but the troponin level is slightly elevated. What is the probability that this patient is having a myocardial infarction?

At first glance, the answer to this question seems obvious. Certainly the patient is having a myocardial infarction! Before we jump to this conclusion, however, we must think this through, and we need more information. We need to know the probability that the troponin test will be positive in patients with myocardial infarction, and we need to know something about the patient. Is the diagnosis of myocardial infarction even plausible for this particular patient?

Bayes' Rule

Bayes' Rule was named after The Reverend Thomas Bayes, an English minister who was interested in probability and induction. He wrote an essay, published after he died, in which he proposed a mathematical explanation for conditional probability.

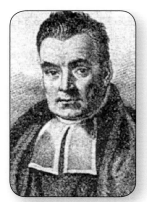
The Reverend Thomas Bayes (1702-1761)

Bayes invented a formula for calculating conditional probability. Using Bayesian logic, we calculate conditional probabilities by first estimating a baseline probability and then revising the probability based on new information. Depending on the strength of the new information, our initial probability estimate may be changed a lot or a little. Bayes' Rule helps us put a number on conditional probability and adjust our thinking based on new information. It provides a way to objectively learn from experience.

The conditional probability of A given B is defined as p(A&B)/p(B). Using this definition, we can derive Bayes' Rule, as shown in Sidebar 3.2. In step 1, we use the notation p(A|B), which means "the probability of A, given B." Rather than using the terms A and B, in this example we will substitute terms that pertain to medicine. In step 2, we change the notation from p(A|B) to p(D|+), which means the probability of having the disease (e.g., myocardial infarction), given a positive test (e.g., troponin).

Step 3 simply states that the probability of a positive test is the sum of the true-positive rate and the false-positive rate. Step 4 combines Step 2 and Step 3.

Step 5 restates the definition of conditional probability for patients without disease. Step 6 rearranges terms and Step 7 combines terms to yield the Bayes' Rule.

Step 8 replaces some of the terms with terms that are more familiar. The term p(+|D) is the true positive rate, or the sensitivity, and the term p(+|~D) is the false positive rate, or 1-the specificity.

In Step 9, we put in actual numbers for a high-sensitivity troponin test. For troponin, the sensitivity is 0.95 and the specificity is 0.80. If, for example, we assume that our prior probability estimate is 0.50, we can use the formula to calculate

Sidebar 3.2 Derivation of Bayes' Rule. [p(A|B) = the probability of A, given B, D = patients with disease, ~D = patients without disease.]

1. Definition: $p(A|B) = \dfrac{p(A \text{ and } B)}{p(B)}$

2. Definition: $p(D|+) = \dfrac{p(+ \text{ and } D)}{p(+)}$

3. $p(+) = p(+ \text{ and } D) + p(+ \text{ and } \sim D)$

4. Thus $p(D|+) = \dfrac{p(+ \text{ and } D)}{p(+ \text{ and } D) + p(+ \text{ and} \sim D)}$

5. Definition: $p(+|\sim D) = \dfrac{p(+ \text{ and } \sim D)}{p(\sim D)}$

6. Rearranging:

   $p(+ \text{ and } \sim D) = p(\sim D) \times p(+|\sim D)$

7. Combining:

   $p(D|+) = \dfrac{p(D) \times p(+|D)}{p(D) \times p(+|D) + p(\sim D) \times p(+|\sim D)}$

8. $p(D|+) = \dfrac{p(D) \times TPR}{p(D) \times TPR + p(\sim D) \times FPR}$

9. $p(D|+) = \dfrac{.5 \times .95}{.5 \times .95 + .5 \times .2} = .83$

that the post test probability of myocardial infarction given a positive troponin is 0.83.

Bayes' Rule gives us a way to shift our thinking from an initial impression to a final impression, based on a positive or negative test result, as shown in Figure 3.11. Bayes' Rule provides a way to incorporate the operating characteristics of the test (i.e., the sensitivity and the specificity) into our probabilistic assessment of the patient.

Figure 3.12 shows how we can apply this method to a particular patient. We can choose a prior probability from the range of prior probabilities on the x-axis. Let's choose 0.50. We can draw a line up from the 0.50 point to the points on the curves for a positive test and a negative test, and then draw a line to the y-axis to determine the posterior probability. As shown, the shift in probability is much greater for a patient with a mid-range prior probability. For patients with very low or very high prior probabilities, the test result has much less effect on our posttest thinking. For patients with either very low or very high pretest probabilities of disease, it makes little sense to perform a test because the test result, if we are thinking correctly, should have little influence on our estimate of posttest probability. A common mistake is to take the test

Figure 3.11 Shifting our thinking from a prior probability to a posterior probability based on either a positive or negative test result.

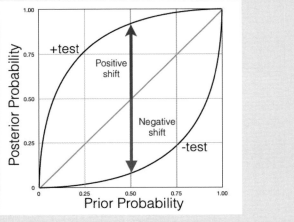

Figure 3.12 Shifting our thinking based on either a positive or negative test result.

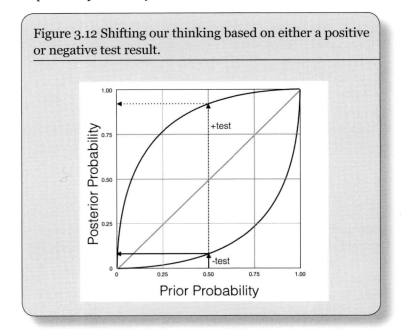

result as the final answer, without proper regard for the prior probability estimate.

In clinical practice, we usually don't formally calculate posttest probabilities, even though we have smartphones and computers at our fingertips. You would think that we would just pull out our smartphones and calculate the probabilities. We don't, and I don't think it is because doctors are just lazy. I suspect that doctors have an intuitive sense that exact calculations may have a false precision. Perhaps we realize that the prior probabilities are somewhat imprecise estimates that would yield equally imprecise posttest probabilities. Perhaps we also realize that the posttest probabilities don't give us a categorical yes-or-no answer. We would still have to set an arbitrary threshold or cutoff to turn a probability estimate into a categorical answer.

Anchoring and Adjusting Heuristic

Rather than using calculated probabilities, we tend to use a heuristic, or mental process, called anchoring and adjusting. With anchoring and adjusting, we intuitively estimate the prior probability, which we call the anchor, and then intuitively adjust the probability estimate based on new information. Rather than turning the process over to a calculator or computer, human nature has taught us to perform the process intuitively.

Anchoring and adjusting is used frequently, rapidly, and usually effectively. Anchoring and adjusting can, however, lead to two types of error: anchoring and base-rate neglect. Anchoring is simply getting too stuck on the initial impression of prior probability and not making the appropriate adjustment. Base-rate neglect occurs when we forget about the prior probability and take the test result at face value.

The example in Sidebar 3.3 shows the problem of base-rate neglect.[4] A witness saw a cab sideswipe another car on a foggy night. Even though the witness reported that it was a blue cab, it is still more likely that the sideswiping cab was a green cab, given that 85% of the cabs in town are green and the witness has a 20% error rate.

A medical example of base-rate neglect is frequently mentioned in the cognitive psychology literature and has been called the "Harvard Medical School Problem." This example comes from an interesting article published in 1978 in the New England Journal of Medicine by Ward Casscells.[5]

In this study, Dr. Casscells asked 60 of his colleagues at a Harvard teaching hospital the following question:

"If a test to detect a disease whose prevalence is one in a thousand has a false-positive rate of 5%, what is the chance that a person found to have a positive result actually has the disease, assuming that you know nothing about the person's symptoms or signs?"

Only 18% of these Harvard doctors gave the correct answer. Forty-five percent said 95%! As shown in Table 3.1, the correct

One night a cab sideswiped another car. A witness saw the event and said it was a blue cab.

All the cabs in town are either blue or green. 85% are green.

It was a foggy night. Under similar conditions, the witness was found to be correct 80% of the time.

Was the sideswiper most likely a blue or a green cab?

Answer: 68% chance it was green despite the witness' testimony (0.85 x 0.8 =0.68).

the doctors assumed that the two rates were complementary probabilities. This mistake is a form of denominator neglect, or losing track of the terms in the denominator. They failed to recognize that the false-positive rate and the positive predictive value have different denominators.

Cognitive psychologists tell us that we can improve how we handle probability problems and avoid both base-rate neglect and denominator neglect by expressing the probabilities using natural frequencies rather than percentages. There is a theory that we are better equipped to use natural frequencies rather than percentages because we evolved using natural frequencies and have been using them since primitive times. We therefore find natural frequencies much more intuitive. When we use percentages, we tend to lose track of the reference class, leading to confusion and miscalculations, and this can happen even to smart Harvard doctors.

To test this theory, the cognitive psychologists Cosmides and Tooby gave the identical problem to 25 Stanford students.[6] First they repeated the problem by asking the same question, and they found that Stanford students were no better than the Harvard doctors. Only 12% gave the correct answer. Then the investigators asked the question using natural frequencies: "One in a thousand people have a certain disease. A test can detect the disease well, but out of 1000 people without the disease, 50 will test positive. What is the probability that a person with a positive test actually has the disease?"

Asked this way, 75% got the correct answer. Using natural frequencies was more intuitive. Using natural frequencies

answer is 1 out of 51, or 2%. Most of the Harvard doctors gave a much higher number, clearly committing base-rate neglect. The doctors who guessed 95% just got confused by the numbers. They were given the false-positive rate of 5% and were asked the positive predictive value. Apparently,

Table 3.1 The "Harvard Medical School Problem"[5]

	PRESENT	**ABSENT**	
Test +	1	50	51
Test -	0	949	949
	1	999	1000

enabled the respondents to keep track of the reference classes of the probabilities used in the question. Percentages help us make comparisons by normalizing to a common denominator (100), but when we use percentages, sometimes we lose track of what the denominator represents.

Using natural frequencies can help us make better intuitive estimates of prior and posttest probabilities. Using natural frequencies can help us discuss probability with patients and families more clearly. Even better, we can use pictorial representations of natural frequencies to help laypeople grasp the meaning of probabilities like operative risk.

In everyday practice, we use anchoring and adjusting intuitively and almost unconsciously. This intuitive approach can be improved if we recalibrate our intuition from time to time. We can calibrate our intuition by checking our estimates of prior probability against some reference like an observational study, or objective measurement of our own aggregated experience. We can use likelihood ratios to calibrate the magnitude of our adjustment in our anchoring and adjusting heuristics. Briefly, a likelihood ratio gives us a measure of the weight of a new piece of evidence. We can multiply the prior odds of some event or proposition by the likelihood ratio to calculate the posttest odds. This is easy enough to do in our heads. (We will cover this thoroughly in the next chapter.)

There are nomograms that help us determine posttest probability of a diagnosis from the prior probability and the

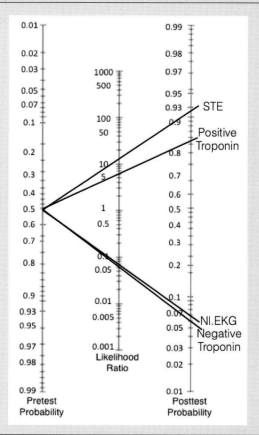

Figure 3.13. Nomogram showing how likelihood ratios for ST elevation or a normal EKG and for a positive or a negative single troponin test can change the post test probability of acute myocardial infarction.

likelihood ratios. A nomogram provides a good visual rendering of how anchoring and adjusting works. As shown in Figure 3.13, we can anchor our prior probability of a patient having an acute myocardial infarction, say at 0.5, on the scale to the left of the figure. We then draw a straight line across the middle scale, which shows the likelihood ratios, in this case for an initial electrocardiogram and for a high-sensitivity troponin test. The likelihood ratios are indicators of the strength of the new evidence provided by the electrocardiogram and the troponin test. We continue the line to the scale at the right, which shows the posttest probability of acute myocardial infarction.

The nomogram example shows how we anchor our initial probability estimate, and we adjust the estimate based on new evidence. As we can see, the EKG result should strongly affect our thinking. With ST-segment elevation, the probability shifts from 0.5 to 0.92. With a normal EKG, the posttest probability shifts from 0.5 to 0.07. Our posttest probability changes fairly dramatically depending on the EKG result.

In a similar fashion, a single troponin test, whether positive or negative, can dramatically shift our thinking about a patient with suspected myocardial infarction. A positive troponin shifts our probability estimate to 0.82, whereas a negative troponin shifts our probability estimate to 0.06–a fairly substantial change from the prior probability of 0.5 that we used for an anchor. The nomogram example presented here is a graphic rendering of how we use the anchoring and adjusting heuristic.

Recalibrating our Intuitive Approaches

The work of our profession demands that we develop an intuitive sense and a deep understanding of probability, which is critical for sound inductive reasoning in everyday practice. We use these skills whenever we estimate the chances of a diagnosis or predict an outcome. Good diagnostic and prognostic estimates are essential as we aim to choose optimal treatment strategies for our patients.

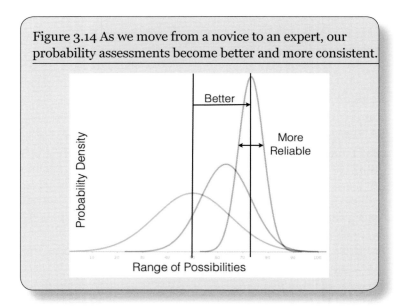

Figure 3.14 As we move from a novice to an expert, our probability assessments become better and more consistent.

As we gain experience during our careers, our probability estimates improve (Figure 3.14). We increase our accuracy (our estimates get closer to the mark) and our precision (we achieve greater reliability and consistency). In short, we "get it

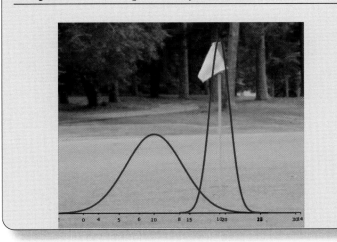

Figure 3.15 As we gain expertise, we gain both accuracy and precision in our probability estimates.

right" more frequently and with less variability (Figure 3.15). With years of training and with the benefit of the example of senior experts, our wild guesses are replaced by more-plausible hypotheses. An emphasis on medical reasoning during early training fosters the crucial, lifelong habit of honing our intuitive skills deliberately and persistently.

Also, experts with extensive experience need to recalibrate their intuitive sense of probability from time to time. Objective feedback from peers and colleagues, as well as continuing medical education that includes refresher courses on probability, can help in that effort. By periodically recalibrating our probability estimates, we can avoid a drift in judgment and bolster our ability to stay true to the mark.

The next chapter discusses how we use conditional probability, Bayesian logic, likelihood ratios, and the anchoring and adjusting heuristic to make medical decisions.

References:

1. Hacking I. An introduction to probability and inductive logic. Cambridge, U.K.; New York: Cambridge University Press; 2001.

2. Hacking I. The taming of chance. Cambridge England; New York: Cambridge University Press; 1990.

3. Keynes JM. A Treatise on Probability. London: Macmillan & Co.; 1921.

4. Kahneman D. Thinking, fast and slow. New York: Farrar, Straus and Giroux; 2011.

5. Casscells W, Schoenberger A, Graboys TB. Interpretation by physicians of clinical laboratory results. The New England Journal of Medicine. 1978; 299:999-1001

6. Cosmides L, Tooby J. Are humans good intuitive statisticians after all? Cognition. 1996;58(1):1-73.

Chapter 4

Decision Making: Making Choices

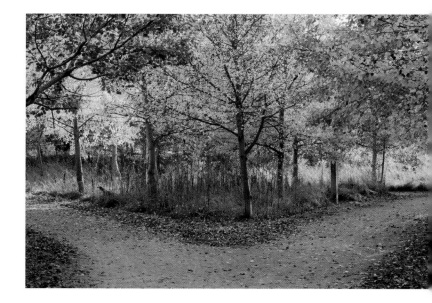

The first order of business when solving a problem is to ask, "What is the nature of the problem?" Herbert Simon, the father of cognitive psychology and artificial intelligence, defined two fundamental types of problems: structured decisions and unstructured problems.[1] Decision making is a structured process—a simple choice. Unstructured problems, in contrast, are problems that are solved by more-complex mental processes. This chapter will cover structured decisions and the use of conditional probabilities, Bayesian logic, likelihood ratios, and the anchoring and adjusting heuristic. Unstructured decisions will be the topic of the next chapter.

Let's return to the example of a woman who comes to the emergency room reporting chest pain. The pain is now gone. The EKG is normal. A troponin level is slightly elevated. Does this patient have a myocardial infarction or not? The answer depends on the attributes of the test and on the situation, but the decision has some structure. The structure allows us to use reasoning and to apply probability rules to make the decision. Knowledge of the test characteristics and of how to use the test properly allows us to immediately start solving the problem.

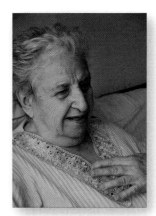

A structured decision is a simple choice. The choice in this case is whether to accept or reject the proposition that this patient is having an acute myocardial infarction. The answer depends on some baseline characteristics of the patient in question and on the operating characteristics of the troponin test.

A patient comes to the emergency room with chest pain. The troponin is slightly elevated.

Operating Characteristics of a Clinical Test
A typical test is a laboratory measurement that reports results on a continuous scale. A group of random people has a range of possible values for the measurement, and the limits of the normal range are determined statistically, usually within two standard deviations from the mean value (Figure 4.1). This works very well for a laboratory test like a serum sodium level, although this approach does create a problem when a clinician orders a battery of lab tests as a screening procedure. With a shotgun approach like a battery of tests, one of the tests is statistically likely to fall out of the normal range, giving a false-positive result.

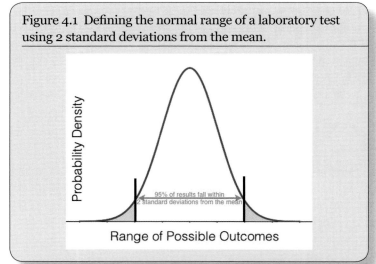

Figure 4.1 Defining the normal range of a laboratory test using 2 standard deviations from the mean.

Simply defining a statistical normal range, and reporting as abnormal any lab results outside that range, may not be appropriate for a test like a troponin level. Troponin is a marker of myocardial injury, so normal people should not have any circulating troponin. Also, confounding conditions other than myocardial infarction, such as sepsis or renal failure, can cause a troponin elevation, so interpreting troponin tests can be tricky.

Nevertheless, the designers of any test have to decide where on the x-axis to draw the line of demarcation defining test results as normal or abnormal. As shown in Figure 4.2, a line of demarcation is like a partition. It defines the test results on one side of the line as normal and the test results on the other side of the line as abnormal. The designers of the test try to draw the line at a point that maximizes the test's usefulness. As shown in Figure 4.3, if the line is moved to the right, more patients without disease are included, and the test becomes more specific. However, this comes at a cost of creating more false-negative results, as shown in the middle panel of Figure 4.3. If the line is moved to the left, more patients with disease are included, and the test becomes more sensitive. This also comes at a cost of creating more false-positive results, as shown in the lower panel of Figure 4.3.

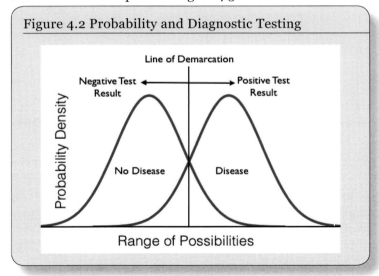

Figure 4.2 Probability and Diagnostic Testing

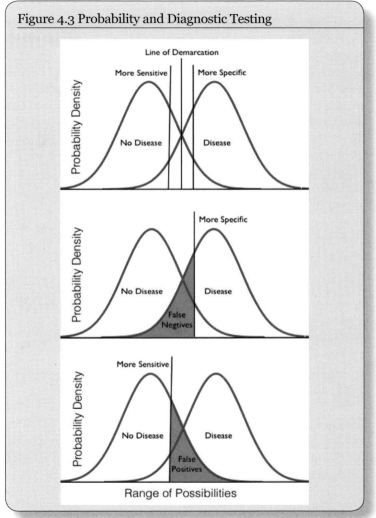

Figure 4.3 Probability and Diagnostic Testing

In the case of troponin, the line has been placed to maximize sensitivity. A panel of experts has recommended setting the cut-point for troponin at the 99th percentile of values for a normal reference group. This cut-point actually defines a very high specificity, not sensitivity, but because most normal people have no detectable troponin, the 99th percentile for a normal reference group is an extremely low level and this low cut-point also happens to define a very high sensitivity. New high-sensitivity assays can precisely measure troponin at these low levels.[2] An international consensus panel has stipulated additional criteria for diagnosing acute myocardial infarction.[3] This definition stipulates that a patient must have a typical rise and fall of the troponin level and that the test must be performed in an appropriate clinical setting. This definition largely excludes false-positive troponin elevations that arise from confounding conditions such as renal failure.

The characteristics of a clinical test, shown in Table 4.1, are determined through clinical research. Investigators identify the frequencies of positive and negative test results among patients known to have disease and among people known to be normal, as determined by a gold-standard test. From the frequencies of the test results, the investigators can calculate the test's sensitivity and specificity, as shown in Table 4.1.

The sensitivity of the test is the proportion of patients with a disease who have a positive test. It is the **true positive rate:** TP/(TP + FN). In Table 4.1, it is the number in cell A divided by the number in cell G.

The specificity of the test is the proportion of patients without disease who have a negative test. It is the **true negative rate:** TN/(TN + FP). In Table 4.1, it is the number in cell E divided by the number in cell H.

Table 4.1 Characteristics of a test.

	TRUE STATE OF THE PATIENT		
	+ Disease	- Disease	
+ Test	A TP	B FP	C + Test
-Test	D FN	E TN	F - Test
	G +Disease	H -Disease	Total Population

Sensitivity=A/G, Specificity=E/H, Positive Predictive Value=A/C, Negative Predictive Value=E/F

A perfect test reflects complete separation between patients with and those without disease. Unfortunately, perfect tests are extremely rare in medicine. The test results of patients with disease and those of patients without disease usually overlap substantially.

Figure 4.4 shows probability density curves (blue) for

patients with disease and with no disease. The cumulative probability curves (red) have been added to show the true positive rates (TPR, or sensitivity) and the true negative rates (TNR, or specificity), depending on where we place the line of demarcation.

Figure 4.4 Probability density curves (blue) for patients with disease and with no disease and the corresponding cumulative probability curves (red) for the true positive rates (TPR, or sensitivity) and the true negative rates (TNR, or specificity), depending on where we draw the line of demarcation.

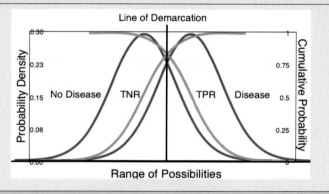

In the top panel of Figure 4.5, we have taken the TPR and TNR curves from Figure 4.4 and we have added a cumulative probability curve (shown in black) for the false positive rate (FPR), which is the complimentary probability of the true negative rate (1-specificity). From the TPR and the FPR

Figure 4.5 Plotting the TPR ("the signal") on the y-axis and the FPR ("the noise") on the x-axis to create an ROC curve. Three sample coordinates are shown in purple, black and blue and are plotted to form the ROC curve below.

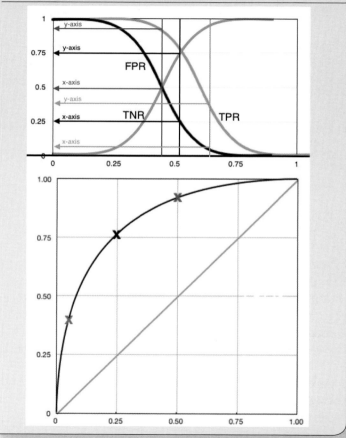

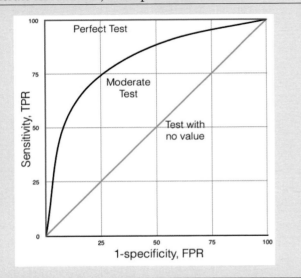

Figure 4.6 ROC Curve: the true positive rate versus the false positive rate. The figure shows a test with no value in red, a moderate test in black, and a perfect test in blue.

the TPR curve and the x-coordinates off the FPR curve. The resulting plot of the TPR and FPR at various discrimination thresholds would yield the black curve in the lower panel of Figure 4.5 and in Figure 4.6.

For a worthless test, the signal and noise probability curves are superimposed. A test that can't separate signal from noise has no value. The line comparing the cumulative probability curves of signal and noise is a straight diagonal with a slope of 1, as shown by the red line in Figure 4.6.

The plot of signal and noise for a moderate test is shown by the black curve in Figure 4.6. A good test with high sensitivity and specificity has an ROC curve that is convex upward. The area under the curve (AUC, or the "c-statistic") is a measure of how good the test is. A better test has a higher c-statistic, and a perfect test has a c-statistic of 1.

A perfect test completely separates the signal from the noise, as shown in Figure 4.7. In the figure, the cumulative probability value for the signal rises to the maximum before the cumulative probability value of the noise starts to rise. Thus, the plot of signal to noise for a perfect test is a line that rises all the way up the y-axis before moving down the x-axis, as shown by the blue line in Figure 4.6.

ROC curves were developed by the radio industry to evaluate how well a radio separates signal from noise. When we try to distinguish patients with disease from patients without disease, we are essentially trying to separate signal from

cumulative probability curves, we can create another graph by plotting the true-positive rate (the "signal") on the y-axis and the false-positive rate (the "noise") on the x-axis to produce something called a receiver operating characteristic (ROC) curve, as shown in the lower panel in Figure 4.5 and in Figure 4.6.

Figure 4.5 shows how we can plot an ROC curve. Imagine taking a vertical line of demarcation and sweeping it from right to left in the top graph, reading the y-coordinates off

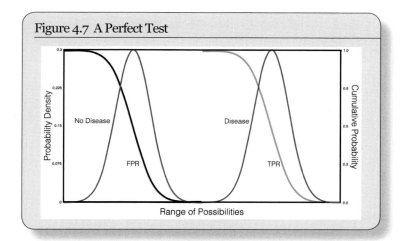

Figure 4.7 A Perfect Test

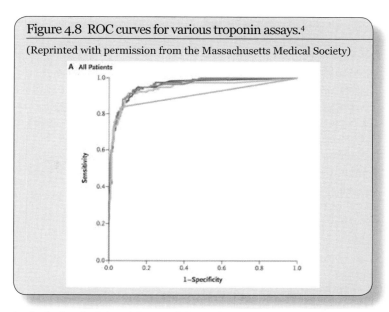

Figure 4.8 ROC curves for various troponin assays.[4]

(Reprinted with permission from the Massachusetts Medical Society)

noise, making ROC curves a good tool for evaluating medical diagnostic tests. ROC curves plot the true-positive rate versus the false-positive rate at various discrimination thresholds.

The ROC curves for various high-sensitivity troponin assays are shown in Figure 4.8.[4] The c-statistic is 0.92, indicating that the test is a good one. The test has a sensitivity (true positive rate) of 95% and a specificity (true negative rate) of 80%.

The operating characteristics of any test are developed in a research setting where investigators measure the ability of the test to detect a diagnosis in a population of patients with disease and reject the diagnosis in a population of people without disease. The spectrum of patients included in the research study can affect the measured operating characteristics of the test. For example, if a study population included only "the sickest of the sick," the research may show that a test is quite sensitive. If one expects the same operating characteristics for a test in practice, the test must be used in a similar spectrum of patients. If the test is used in practice on a different spectrum of patients, the operating characteristics of the test may change (a phenomenon called "spectrum bias"). For example, consider the specificity and sensitivity of high-sensitivity troponin testing defined in a population that excludes patients with renal failure. If the test is used clinically in a population that includes the confounding diagnosis of renal failure, there is a higher rate of false-positive results, yielding a lower specificity. To avoid spectrum bias, a test must be used in the proper clinical setting.

Test Ordering Strategies

Another problem arises when tests are used indiscriminately in a broad range of patients. Such over-testing can also yield a large number of false positives. Screening strategies are subject to this problem. When we use a test to screen a large number of patients with a very low prior probability of a diagnosis, it is hard to find a line of demarcation that will prevent the inclusion of a large number of patients without disease. As shown in Figure 4.9, the number of patients without disease and a positive test (false positives) can substantially exceed the number of patients with disease who are correctly identified (true positives).

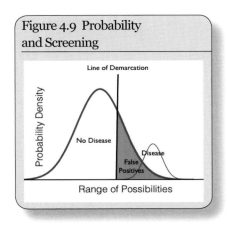

Figure 4.9 Probability and Screening

To illustrate this further, Figure 4.10 shows how troponin testing works over the long run in a population of 1000 patients with a 1% prior probability of acute myocardial infarction. Because of the low prior probability, the positive predictive value (the posttest probability, given a positive test) is only 4%. Positive predictive value is the number of patients with a true-positive result divided by the total number of patients

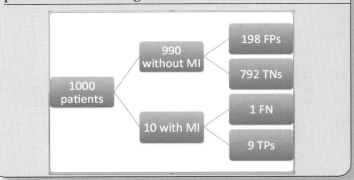

Figure 4.10 Applying a troponin test with 95% sensitivity and 80% specificity to a population with a prior probability of 1% yields a positive predictive value of only 4% (9 TPs/9 TPs +198 FPs). The odds are 96 to 4, or 24 to 1 against a positive test result being correct.

with a positive test result, in this case 9/(9 + 198). Because of the low prior probability, the odds are 24 to 1 against a positive result being correct. Believing a positive result in this case would be making a very bad bet.

Now consider a second example: A series of patients with a 25% prior probability of acute myocardial infarction undergo troponin testing (Figure 4.11). Here the positive predictive value is 61% (238/[238 + 150]), a far more helpful result. The true positives outnumber the false positives 1.5 to 1. Believing a positive result in this case would be a reasonable bet. So the way to combat excessive false-positive test results is to use testing judiciously.

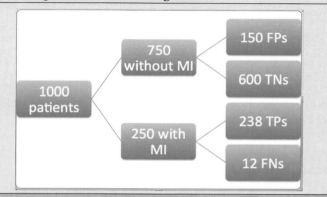

In these two examples, we have used a frequency notion of probability to imagine how troponin testing would turn out over the long run in two populations with defined pretest probabilities. When we order a troponin test, however, we are ordering the test for a single patient. To think about a single person, we need to switch to the personal notion of probability. We must think about how a troponin test result would shift our belief about the probability of an acute myocardial infarction in single patient.

As shown in Figure 4.12, a positive troponin in a patient with a prior probability of 1% should have very little effect on our thinking. The shift in our belief about the posttest probability

is so small that it is barely visible in the lower left corner of the graph. There is a much greater shift in our thinking with a patient whose prior probability is 25%, as shown in Figure 4.12.

Figure 4.12 Personal notion of probability applied to a troponin test showing how a positive test will shift our thinking from a prior probability of 1% (in yellow) or 25% (in blue).

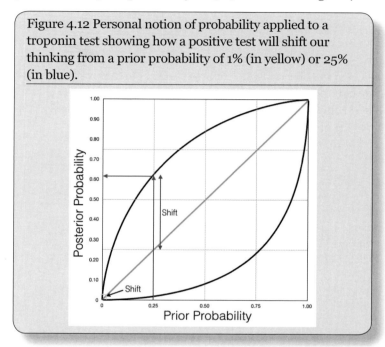

Whether you view testing strategies as a frequentist or as a Bayesian, it is obvious that tests like troponin are best used in patients with mid-range prior probabilities. When using testing at the extreme ends of the range of prior probabilities, the test result should not shift our probability estimate very much, if we are thinking properly. These examples show that ordering the test for patients with extremely low or extremely high prior probabilities is a misleading, useless exercise.

To further illustrate this point, consider some examples of stress testing to diagnose coronary artery disease. For optimal use of stress testing, the ordering physician must have some idea of the prior probability of coronary artery disease. We are greatly helped in this regard by a classic paper, published in 1979, that gives us an estimate of prior probability of coronary artery disease according to gender, age, and type of presenting symptoms.[5] The results of this paper are summarized in Table 4.2.

Table 4.2 Prior probability of coronary artery disease from Diamond and Forrester.[5]						
	NON- ANGINAL CHEST PAIN		ATYPICAL ANGINA		TYPICAL ANGINA	
Age	Men	Women	Men	Women	Men	Women
30-39	5.2	0.8	21.8	4.2	68.7	25.8
40-49	14.1	2.8	46.1	13.3	87.3	55.2
50-59	21.4	8.4	58.9	32.4	92.0	79.4
60-69	28.1	18.6	67.1	54.4	94.3	90.6

Although reports in the literature vary, imaging stress testing typically has a sensitivity of 90% and a specificity of 85%. These characteristics can vary by laboratory, and some evidence suggests that stress echocardiography has a slightly higher specificity and a lower sensitivity than nuclear stress testing does. Also, an interpreting physician may systematically over-read the images, thereby ramping up the sensitivity and ramping down the specificity. By the same token, an interpreting physician may under-read the images, with the opposite effect on sensitivity and specificity. Nevertheless, the general estimates of sensitivity and specificity for imaging stress tests are 90% and 85%. Given these imperfect test characteristics, we can see that it is a bad idea to use the tests in patients with extremely high or extremely low prior probabilities of coronary artery disease.

Let's use an example of a 65-year-old man with typical angina. We can look up his prior probability in Table 4.2 and find that it is 94%. As shown in Figure 4.13, if we had a thousand similar patients and put them all through imaging stress testing with a sensitivity of 90% and specificity of 85%, we would generate these results: 9 false positives, 51 true negatives, 94 false negatives, and 846 true positives. A negative test result doesn't really help us here because it is almost twice as likely to be wrong rather than right. It would be a big mistake to believe a negative test result in this case. If, for some reason, you harbor doubts about the diagnosis in a patient with a prior probability of 94%, stress testing wouldn't give you strong enough evidence to reject the diagnosis. A cardiac catheterization might be necessary for definitive evaluation.

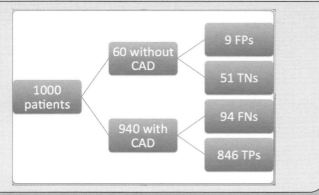

Figure 4.13 Imaging stress testing in a population with a prior probability of CAD of 94% yields a false negative rate of 65% (94/94+51). In this population, the odds are 65 to 35, or almost 2 to 1 against a negative test result being correct.

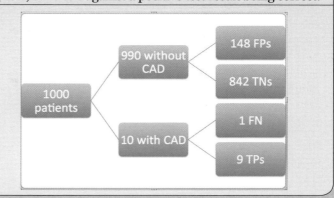

Figure 4.14 Imaging stress testing in a population with a prior probability of CAD of 1% yields a positive predictive value of only 6% (9/9+148). In this population, the odds are 94 to 6, or 16 to 1 against a positive test result being correct.

Another example is a 39-year-old woman with non-anginal chest pain. We can look up her prior probability in Table 4.2 and find that it is just less than 1%. As shown in Figure 4.14, if we had a thousand similar patients and performed imaging stress testing, we would generate 148 false-positive tests for every 9 true-positive tests. The posttest probability, given a positive test, would be only 6%. In this case, a positive test result is misleading: It is 16 times more likely to be wrong rather than right. It would be a big mistake to believe a positive test result in this case. Most likely, the positive test result would result in a cardiac catheterization for definitive evaluation.

The better strategy is to avoid stress testing in a patient with such a low prior probability, unless you are prepared to deal with a false-positive test. Indiscriminate testing leads to a diagnostic cascade of more testing with added expense, unnecessary radiation exposure, and a fixed (albeit a low) rate of cath-lab complications.

Again, we can switch our thinking about these examples from the frequentist to the personal notion of probability, as shown in Figure 4.15. For our patient whose prior probability of coronary artery disease is 94%, we see that a negative imaging stress test will shift our thinking about the patient, but the posttest probability remains above 50%. If we analyze the test

Figure 4.15 Personal notion of probability applied to an imaging stress test showing how a negative test will shift our thinking from a prior probability of 95% (in blue) and how a positive test will shift our thinking from a prior probability of 1% (in yellow).

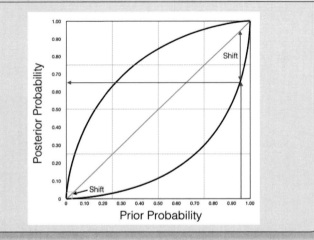

result properly, the shift in our thinking should not be enough to change our minds about whether the patient has coronary artery disease. For the patient with a prior probability of 1%, a positive stress test should yield a negligible shift in our thinking, one so small that it is barely visible in the lower left corner of Figure 4.15.

The problem of screening a low-risk population also applies to other tests, including mammography and prostate-specific antigen (PSA) testing. For cancer screening, there is an

Sidebar 4.1 Problems with screening and survival rates.

Proponents of cancer screening point to improved survival rates to argue in favor of cancer screening strategies. Gigerenzer, however, shows us that there is a fundamental flaw in this reasoning.[6] He demonstrates this flaw with a statement made in the popular press by Rudy Giuliani about prostate cancer. Giuliani claimed, "I had prostate cancer 5 or 6 years ago. My chance of surviving prostate cancer - and thank God, I was cured of it - in the United States? Eighty-two percent. My chance of surviving prostate cancer in England? Only 44 percent under socialized medicine."

Was Rudy Giuliani right? Are we really that much better at treating prostate cancer in the U.S. than in England? The answer is obviously no. His statistics were correct, but his conclusions were wrong. He was referring to the 5-year survival rates for the year 2000. That year in the U.S., most prostate cancer was detected by prostate-specific antigen (PSA) testing, whereas in the U.K., most prostate cancer was detected by symptoms. That created a lead-time bias for the U.S, as shown in the figure.

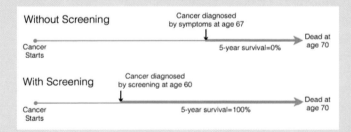

PSA testing also led to the detection of many non-progressive cancers. The fact is that in 2000 the mortality rates for prostate cancer was virtually identical in the U.S. and the U.K. (26/100,000 versus 27/100,000). So there are many reasons to be skeptical and cautious about strategies of screening for disease.

additional consideration. It is possible that the screening test will find an abnormality that is actually a low-level cancer that is unlikely to alter a patient's long-term outcome. Problems with cancer screening and survival rates are discussed in Sidebar 4.1.

The best strategy for ordering diagnostic testing is to use the Bayesian logic discussed in the previous chapter. As discussed, we typically replace a numerical Bayesian calculation with a heuristic known as anchoring and adjusting. We seem to prefer intuitive approaches to formal calculations using Bayes' Rule. We can improve our Bayesian approach and our use of anchoring and adjusting by using likelihood ratios. Likelihood ratios can help us calibrate our intuitive use of the anchoring and adjusting heuristic.

Likelihood Ratios

Likelihood is an idea proposed by the R.A. Fisher, often considered the father of modern statistics. Likelihood sounds as though it ought to be synonymous with probability, but Fisher defined likelihood in a very technical way: p(E|H), or the probability of gaining some evidence (i.e., getting some test result), given that a hypothesis (i.e., the presence of disease) is true. Fisher's idea of likelihood helps us define a very helpful tool: the likelihood ratio.

A likelihood ratio is the percentage of diseased people with a given test result divided by the percentage of well people with the same test result. It is a ratio of probabilities. The likelihood ratio is handy because we can multiply the likelihood ratio[7,8]

times the prior odds (also a ratio of probabilities) to yield the posttest odds. A likelihood ratio offers a simple and intuitive way to understand the capability of a test. This objective estimate of a test's validity can give us a better idea of how to use that test in our anchoring and adjusting heuristic. How much weight should we give to this new piece of evidence? The positive likelihood ratio for a positive test result and the negative likelihood ratio for a negative test result can offer a general idea of the weight of the evidence. More information about likelihood ratios is presented in Appendix 2.

A positive likelihood ratio is the probability of a positive test result in diseased persons divided by the probability of a positive test result in non-diseased persons: the true-positive rate (TPR) divided by the false-positive rate (FPR). Thus, LR(+) = sensitivity/(1 − specificity). (You may remember that, earlier, we plotted this relation between the TPR and the FPR in our ROC curves.)

For a high-sensitivity troponin test with a sensitivity of 95% and specificity of 80%, the LR(+) = 0.95/(1 − 0.8) = 4.75 (see Table 4.3). For an imaging stress test with a sensitivity of 90% and a specificity of 85%, the LR(+) = 0.9/(1 − 0.85) = 6.0. A test with a likelihood ratio of 1 would be a worthless test. It wouldn't change how you think. A higher LR(+) indicates that the test, if positive, is a stronger signal. A higher LR(+) tells us that a positive test result is a more valid cue and should have a greater influence on your thinking. An LR(+) of 2 to 3 is pretty good. An LR(+) of 10 means that a positive result from that test is a fairly definitive result.

Table 4.3 Likelihood ratios for a troponin test.
LR(+)=TPR/FPR=sensitivity/1-specificity=.95/.2=4.75
LR(-)=FNR/TNR=1-sensitivity/specificity=.05/.8=.06

	MYOCARDIAL INFARCTION		
	+ Disease	- Disease	
+ Troponin	A 95 (0.95)	B 20 (0.2)	C 115
- Troponin	D 5 (0.05)	E 80 (0.8)	F 85
	G 100	H 100	200

The negative likelihood ratio is the probability of a negative test result in diseased persons divided by the probability of a negative test result in non-diseased persons: the false-negative rate (FNR) divided by the true-negative rate (TNR). Thus the LR(-) = (1 − sensitivity)/specificity. The negative likelihood ratio is a fraction, and the lower the better. For our troponin test, the LR(-) = 0.06 (Table 4.3); for our imaging stress test, the LR(-) = 0.12. An LR(-) of 0.5 − 0.3 is pretty good. An LR(-) of 0.1 means that a negative result from that test is fairly definitive.

The likelihood ratio, either the LR(+) or the LR(-), can be multiplied by the prior odds to yield the posttest odds. This is a handy way to calculate the probability of a diagnosis, using a Bayesian-type approach that we can almost compute in

our heads. First, we convert the prior probability to the prior odds, then multiply the odds by the LR to get the posttest odds, and then convert the posttest odds back to probability. Remember that the definition of odds is probability divided by its complementary probability. Converting from probability to odds and back to probability is easy:

Odds = $p/(1 − p)$.

Probability = $odds/(1 + odds)$.

Transforming probability to odds offers some advantages for making calculations, as gamblers know when they calculate the fair payoff of a bet. For instance, if a horse has a 0.75 chance of winning a race, the odds are 0.75/0.25, or 3 to 1 in favor of the horse winning and 1 to 3 that the track will avoid a payoff. A fair payoff for a $3 wager on this horse would be $1. If we try to multiply using probability rather than odds, we get a meaningless result. Consider a patient with a prior probability of coronary artery disease of 75% and a positive test with an LR(+) of 2. Multiplying 75% by 2 yields a posttest probability of coronary artery disease of 150%, which is obviously impossible. By converting the probability into the odds, we covert the number to a form that we can multiply by the likelihood ratios. Other features of odds versus probability are discussed in Sidebar 4.2.

Let's return to our patient whose prior probability of coronary artery disease is 75%. The prior odds are .75/.25 = 3. The prior odds are 3 to 1. Let's say that the LR(-) of some test for CAD

For low values (<0.1), probability and odds are almost equal. This makes sense if we think about the formula for odds: odds=p/1-p. For a low p, the denominator is close to one, making the odds almost equal to the numerator, which is p.

As shown in the panel A, probability has an upper limit of 1.0, but odds has no upper limit. As probability approaches 1.0, odds approaches infinity.

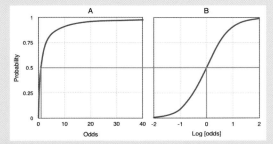

One other interesting point about odds: If we change the odds to the log[odds], the graph of the relation to probability changes into a symmetrical S-shaped curve, with the log[odds] of 0 at the center point of the curve (Panel B). Transforming odds to log[odds] is useful for logistic regression, where the log[odds] is called the logit. We use logistic regression to calculate an outcome variable by adding up multiple predictive variables. The predictive variables can be added after they are transformed to log[odds]. Logistic regression is used to create risk-adjustment models, which will be discussed in Chapter 8.

As shown in the figure, a probability of 0.5 equals an odds of 1.0 and a log[odds] of 0.

Transforming probability to odds and to log[odds] can have many uses.

is 0.33, and the test is negative. The posttest odds are 3 x 0.33 = 1. To convert back to probability, we divide 1 by (1 + 1) = 0.5. Thus, the posttest probability of coronary artery disease in this patient with a negative test result is 50%. A test with an LR(-) of 0.33 shifts our estimate of the probability of CAD from 75% to 50%. A negative test with a LR(-) of 0.33 causes a modest shift in our thinking.

Again, an LR(+) of 2 doubles the odds of an event or proposition. An LR(-) of 0.5 cuts the odds in half. Thus, an LR(+) of 2-3 or an LR(-) of 0.5 − 0.3 starts to indicate that the test result is a valid piece of new information. A test with either an LR(+) or an LR(-) close to 1 is useless and should not influence our thinking.

Of course, likelihood ratios are not exact numbers, given the imprecision in measuring sensitivity and specificity. Figure 4.16 shows how the imprecision of likelihood ratios might determine how a positive or a negative test should affect our thinking. When we say "the positive likelihood ratio is 6," we should probably say, "the positive likelihood ratio is around 6." The likelihood ratios[7,8] of several cardiac tests are listed in Table 4.4. As

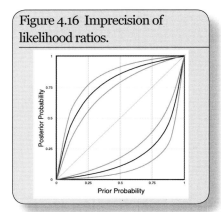

Figure 4.16 Imprecision of likelihood ratios.

shown, some tests are somewhat asymmetric—that is, either the LR(+) or the LR(-) is stronger. For example, a chest X-ray that shows congestion has a very high LR(+). A chest X-ray that is positive for congestion is a very weighty piece of new evidence, whereas a negative chest X-ray is weak evidence. This test should shift your thinking asymmetrically, as shown in Figure 4.17.

Such tests with high specificity are good for "ruling in" a diagnosis, which can be remembered using David Sackett's mnemonic "SpPin" (a test with high specificity that is positive is good for ruling in a diagnosis).[10] Other tests, like BNP or d-dimer, are very sensitive but not very specific. A positive

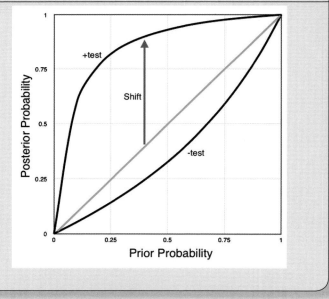

Figure 4.17 Tests with a high specificity and high LR(+) shift our thinking positively and are good for ruling in a diagnosis. This can be remembered with the mnemonic SpPin.

Table 4.4 Likelihood ratios of several cardiac tests.[9] (ER=emergency room, EKG=electrocardiogram, CXR=chest x-ray, CHF=congestive heart failure, BNP=brain natriuretic peptide, PE=pulmonary embolus)

TEST	LR(+)	LR(-)
ST elevation in ER patients with chest pain	11.2	
Normal EKG in ER patients with chest pain		0.07
Single Troponin level	4.75	0.06
Congestion of CXR for CHF	13.5	0.48
Cardiomegaly on CXR for CHF	3.4	0.33
BNP≥100	2.7	0.1
D-dimer for PE	1.7	0.09

d-dimer is a relatively weak piece of evidence, whereas a negative d-dimer is a very weighty piece of new evidence. These tests should also shift our thinking asymmetrically, as shown in Figure 4.18. Such tests with high sensitivity are good for ruling out a diagnosis, which can be remembered using the mnemonic "SnNout" (a test with high sensitivity that is negative is good for ruling out a diagnosis).

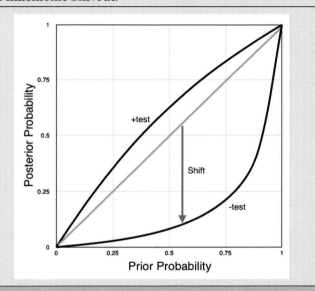

Figure 4.18 Tests with a a high sensitivity and low LR(-) shift our thinking negatively and are good for ruling out a diagnosis. This can be remembered with the mnemonic SnNout.

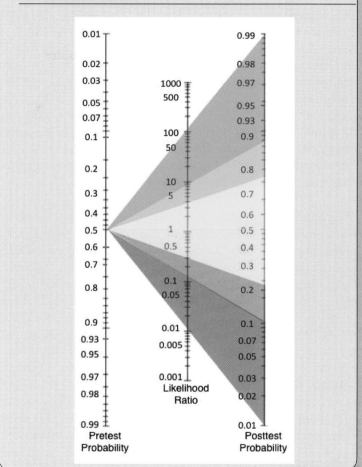

Figure 4.19 Change in probability of a diagnosis depending on the likelihood ratio.

Rather than making the conversion from probability to odds, and then calculating the posttest odds and reconverting back to probability, we can use another readily available tool: nomograms. An example is shown in Figure 4.19.

Nomograms, invented by French engineer Philbert Maurice d'Ocagne in 1884, are frequently used by other engineers, who love precision and accuracy. A nomogram uses scales to make calculations, just like a slide-rule, except that a nomogram's scales don't slide. Instead, the scales are sized and spaced just right, to enable an easy and accurate calculation.

The nomogram for likelihood ratios was first described by Terrence Fagan in a one-page letter to the editor of the New England Journal of Medicine in 1975, long before handheld smartphones existed.[11] In Fagan's nomogram, the pre- and posttest probabilities are on the left and right scales in opposite order, with a probability of 0.5 positioned at the center. The likelihood ratio is on the center scale, with the LR = 1 (having no effect) positioned at the center. Positive likelihood ratios are shown from 1 up on the center scale, negative likelihood ratios from 1 down. The likelihood ratio scale is logarithmic, so the extremes of the scale are compressed.

We can place a straightedge on the left scale at the point of our prior probability estimate and on the center scale at the point of the likelihood ratio, to determine the posttest probability from the scale on the right. The nomogram (Figure 4.19) shows how your impression about a diagnosis would warm up with higher positive likelihood ratios and cool down with lower negative likelihood ratios. A test with a positive likelihood ratio of around 3 represents a solid bit of evidence. One in the 5-7 range is a very solid bit of evidence. A positive result from a test with a positive likelihood ratio greater than 10 is almost pathognomonic. A test with a negative likelihood ratio of less than 0.5 is a solid bit of evidence against a diagnosis. A test with a negative likelihood ratio in the 0.2-0.3 range is more solid and one that is less than 0.1 almost certainly rules out a diagnosis. Remember, that the likelihood ratio is multiplied by the pretest odds to give the posttest odds. To perform the calculation by hand, the pretest probability is converted to odds, multiplied by the likelihood ratio, and posttest odds are converted back to probability. The nomogram does that calculation for you.

The busy practicing clinician doesn't usually pull out a calculator or a nomogram to calculate the probabilities using either Bayes' Rule or likelihood ratios. Stopping to do the calculation would disrupt the clinician's workflow and train of thought. As discussed, we typically use the anchoring and adjusting heuristic. The nomogram does, however, provide a visual rendering of how anchoring and adjusting works.

Although we don't use the hard numbers on a day-to-day basis, we can review hard numbers like likelihood ratios from time to time to calibrate our intuitive judgments. We can calibrate our intuition offline, during reflective moments away from direct patient care, to make sure our judgment doesn't drift from the mark. The nomogram example visually renders the process of anchoring and adjusting. We anchor our initial estimate on the left scale, change our estimate on the basis of new information, and read our adjusted estimate off the right scale. This intuitive Bayesian approach is a sensible method for making structured decisions. Much of medical reasoning, however, is not so structured. Reasoning through unstructured problems is the topic of the next chapter.

References:

1. Simon H. Invariants of human behavior. Annual Review of Psychology. 1990; 41:1-20

2. Newby LK, Jesse RL, Babb JD, Christenson RH, De Fer TM, Diamond GA, Fesmire FM, Geraci SA, Gersh BJ, Larsen GC, Kaul S, McKay CR, Philippides GJ, Weintraub WS. ACCF 2012 expert consensus document on practical clinical considerations in the interpretation of troponin elevations: A report of the American College of Cardiology Foundation task force on clinical expert consensus documents. Journal of the American College of Cardiology. 2012; 60:2427-2463

3. Thygesen K, Alpert JS, Jaffe AS, Simoons ML, Chaitman BR, White HD: the Writing Group on behalf of the Joint ESC/ACCF/AHA/WHF Task Force for the Universal Definition of Myocardial Infarction. Third universal definition of myocardial infarction. Journal of the American College of Cardiology. 2012; 60:1581-1598

4. Reichlin T, Hochholzer W, Bassetti S, Steuer S, Stelzig C, Hartwiger S, Biedert S, Schaub N, Buerge C, Potocki M, Noveanu M, Breidthardt T, Twerenbold R, Winkler K, Bingisser R, Mueller C. Early diagnosis of myocardial infarction with sensitive cardiac troponin assays. The New England journal of medicine. 2009; 361:858-867

5. Diamond GA, Forrester JS. Analysis of probability as an aid in the clinical diagnosis of coronary-artery disease. N Engl J Med. 1979; 300(24): 1350-8.

6. Gigerenzer G, Brighton, H. Homo heuristicus: Why biased minds make better inferences. Topics in Cognitive Science. 2009; 1:107-143

7. Hacking I. Logic of Statistical Inference. Cambridge: Cambridge University Press, 1976.

8. Edwards AWE. Likelihood. Baltimore: The Johns Hopkins University Press, 1992.

9. Simel DL, Rennie D, Keitz SA. The rational clinical examination: Evidence-based clinical diagnosis. New York: McGraw-Hill; 2009.

10. Sackett DL, Haynes RB, Guyatt GH, Tugwell P. Clinical Epidemiology: A Basic Science for Clinical Medicine (Second Edition). Boston: Little, Brown, & Co; 1991.

11. Fagan TJ. Nomogram for Bayes's Theorem. N Engl J Med 1975; 293: 257.

Chapter 5

Solving Unstructured Problems

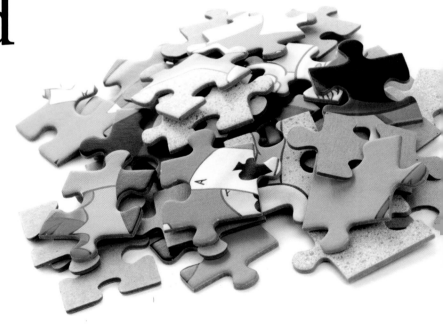

In his analysis of reasoning, Herbert Simon distinguishes between decision making and problem solving, as noted in chapter 4. Decision making is a structured process—a simple choice. Problem solving, in contrast, usually starts out in an unstructured way. To start solving a problem, we must first determine its nature. The initial lack of structure leads us to use heuristics, which are learned mental processes that help us make rapid decisions under conditions of uncertainty. So the fundamental starting point is to determine whether we are dealing with a structured decision or an unstructured problem. If the problem is unstructured, we use a variety of heuristics so that we can start to put the pieces of the puzzle together.

Dealing with uncertainty is like finding your way through darkness. Imagine entering a dark room, maybe your living room, where you have been many times. To find familiar cues, you grope around, perhaps initially encountering a chair that you know is near the door. You use that chair to grope your way to the couch. You feel along the length of the couch to find the end table, where you know a lamp is. You find the lamp and turn on the light. Because the room is familiar, you are

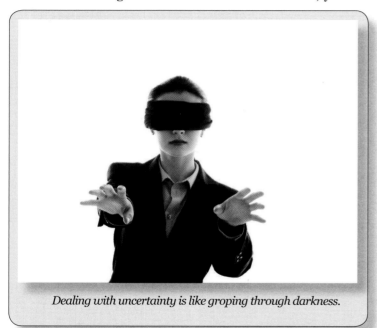
Dealing with uncertainty is like groping through darkness.

able to navigate through the darkness in a purposeful manner to locate the light.

Heuristics are similar. They enable us to navigate through uncertainty with some purpose. Just as experience teaches us how to purposefully grope through darkness in a familiar room, experience teaches us how to use heuristics to deal with uncertainty.

The word heuristic comes from the Greek word "heuriskein," which means "to discover." A heuristic is a mental shortcut. It is an evolved or acquired mental process. Heuristics help us get started with problems by allowing us to gather, process, and organize cues, just as we might arrange and connect disparate dots that together form a whole picture.

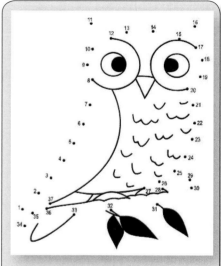
Heuristics help us sort cues to connect the dots, enabling us to imagine the solution to the problem.

The Downside of Heuristics

The question of whether heuristics are good or bad is the subject of considerable debate in the cognitive psychology literature.[1-3] A group led by Daniel Kahneman, a Princeton psychologist and recipient of the Nobel Prize in Economics,[2] has performed many experiments to test how people use heuristics and whether heuristics lead to illogical and inconsistent problem solving. Kahneman and his longtime collaborator Amos Tversky described three heuristics that frequently mislead us: availability, representativeness, and anchoring and adjusting.

The availability heuristic refers to how we are excessively influenced by events that are more recent or more salient than others. These events remain fresh in working memory and crowd out other memories or knowledge that should have greater influence on our thinking.

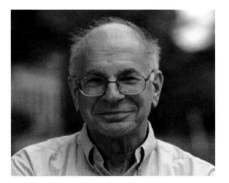

Daniel Kahneman, Cognitive psychologist from Princeton, and recipient of the 2002 Nobel Prize in Economics, argues that heuristics lead to predictable biases and pitfalls.

The representativeness heuristic can cause us to overestimate the probability of an event or a proposition based on appearance or resemblance to something else, without adequately considering the actual probability of the event or proposition. An example is presented in Sidebar 5.1.

According to Kahneman, the anchoring and adjusting heuristic can cause problems. We can become too anchored to our initial probability estimate. Also, priming and bias can misguide where we place the initial anchor. In addition, we

Sidebar 5.1 An example of the representativeness heuristic.

An example of representativeness is an experiment reported by Kahneman and Tversky, which has been called "the Linda problem." They described a hypothetical woman named Linda to experimental subjects and asked the subjects to make a judgment about who Linda was. In the experiment, they described Linda as, "Thirty-one years old, single, outspoken, and very bright. She majored in philosophy. As a student, she was deeply concerned with issues of discrimination and social justice, and also participated in antinuclear demonstrations." They asked their subjects questions like "Is Linda A) a bank teller or B) a bank teller and an activist in the feminist movement?" They found that people were more likely to chose option B. People tended to chose the answer with greater detail, even though the answer was a mistake known as the conjunction fallacy. The probability of multiple attributes occurring simultaneously is less probable that each attribute occurring individually. The responders were attracted to the answer that provided the more detailed description and made a careless error of choosing the less likely choice. These investigators called this tendency the representativeness heuristic.

can forget about the baseline probability and react only to the new information, a problem called base-rate neglect.

With care, we can turn anchoring and adjusting from a weakness into a strength. Done properly, anchoring and adjusting is good Bayesian reasoning. We just have to be careful in estimating the baseline probability and in giving proper weight to the new evidence. Anchoring and adjusting is a useful heuristic that physicians apply every day, notwithstanding Kahneman's view that it is a source of bias.

The heuristics that Kahneman and Tversky describe are failures because they defy the rules of logic or probability. Used improperly, heuristics can cause us to leap to wrong conclusions.

The Upside of Heuristics

Cognitive psychologist Gerd Gigerenzer, of the Max Planck Institute in Berlin, holds an opposing view.[3] He has spent his career evaluating the usefulness of heuristics and believes they evolved for a reason. According to Gigerenzer, rather than rejecting heuristics as flawed, we should embrace them, explore their strengths, and expand their use.

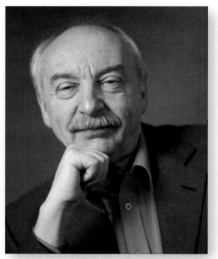

Gerd Gigerenzer, from the Max Plank Institute in Berlin argues that heuristics are highly adaptive and evolved because they are useful.

To support his argument, Gigerenzer refers to the prior work of George Poyla and Herbert Simon. George Poyla (1887–1985), a Hungarian mathematician who spent most of his teaching career at Stanford, wrote a useful and popular introduction to mathematical problem solving called *How to Solve It*.[4] In this book, Polya described the use of heuristics as necessary for starting the task of solving an unstructured problem. He described how heuristics would force the mind to ask the following questions: What is the nature of the problem? What is known? What is unknown? Have I seen anything like this problem before? Is there some analogous or similar problem that I have used before that can help me get started? This type of thinking is not just helpless groping about. It is purposeful because it helps us get a grasp on the problem at hand.

According to Polya, "Heuristic reasoning is not regarded as final and strict, but as provisional and plausible only, whose purpose is to discover the solution to the problem." Polya went on to state "Heuristic reasoning is often based on induction or analogy...What is bad is to mix up heuristic reasoning with rigorous proof." Heuristics provide the initial steps that will ultimately lead to a conclusion.

Herbert Simon extensively investigated how we use heuristics.[5] Like Kahneman, he was the recipient of the Nobel Prize in Economics. Simon's research collaborator for many years was Allen Newell, a student of Polya's at Stanford. Polya introduced the word heuristic to Newell, who then introduced it to Simon.[6]

Herbert Simon coined the term "bounded rationality" to explain that human beings almost never have complete information, unlimited computational ability, or unlimited time to make a decision. Usually, we are bounded by some factors, usually incomplete information. Despite these limitations, we need to act, often rapidly. When we are forced to act under conditions of uncertainty and bounded rationality, we do the best we can under the circumstances, a process that Simon called "satisficing." Rather than optimizing our solutions to problems, we use heuristics and intuition to satisfice. We have to settle for the solution that is just good enough.

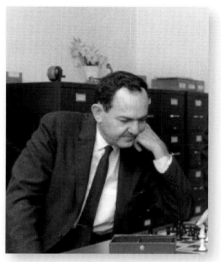

Herbert A. Simon (1916-2001), was the 1978 recipient of the Nobel Prize in Economics and one of the founders of Cognitive Psychology, Behavioral Economics and Artificial Intelligence.

At first, this sounds like an excuse for making sloppy and unnecessary shortcuts. Simon recognized, however, that these shortcuts are strengths, rather than weaknesses, of human nature. Heuristics enable us to move forward and to avoid indecision and analysis paralysis.

Avoiding heuristics is not an option in real-world medical practice. People have held out hope that computers will allow us to eliminate our cognitive shortcuts. The hope is that we can develop artificial intelligence, machine learning, and calculated decision analysis to replace heuristics. People have tried this approach for other applications, such as stock picking and stock-market timing, to no avail. It seems doubtful that we will see the approach successfully adapted for medicine anytime soon. There are too many unknowns, and computer programs can't deal with unknowns. Dealing with unknowns is the forte of heuristics. For solving unstructured clinical problems, even Daniel Kahneman agrees that heuristics are here to stay.[1]

Kahneman is right that heuristics can lead to predictable lapses in thinking. One remedy is to be more attentive to logic and probability.

Gigerenzer uses an analogy, which he calls the gaze heuristic, to explain how heuristics improve decision making (Figure 5.1). To catch a fly ball, a baseball player fixes his gaze on the ball and maintains a constant angle of his

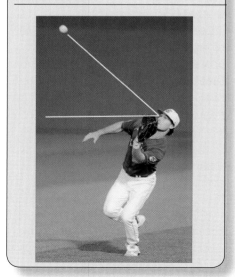

Figure 5.1 The Gaze Heuristic is an analogy that Gerd Gigerenzer uses to explain how "less is more" with heuristics.

gaze by adjusting his running as he maneuvers to catch the ball. If he maintains that constant angle of gaze, he will arrive at just the right place and the ball will fall right into his glove. By using the gaze heuristic, he can ignore the initial distance from the ball, the ball's velocity, the angle from which it was hit, the resistance of the atmosphere, the wind speed, the direction of the ball's spin, and many other variables that might affect the ball's trajectory. Imagine programming a computerized robot to catch a fly ball. Any average little league baseball player can quickly learn this trick and outperform a complicated computerized robot. The gaze heuristic analogy shows us how "less is more" when we use heuristics.

Gigerenzer acknowledges that heuristics have inherent bias, but he argues that this deficiency is offset by heuristics' ability to simplify. Heuristics usually beat out artificial intelligence and machine-learning because they don't fall into the trap of over-fitting noisy information into the decision making process. Computers can create a precise model of the past, but that model may not accurately predict the future. It's like the disclaimer in mutual fund brochures: Past experience is no guarantee of future performance. Philosopher David Hume warned us about this 300 years ago, as discussed in Chapter 2. Computerized predictions typically fail because they incorporate extra data into predictive models that lack any predictive value. The algorithms can't completely filter out the noise. Computers can outperform heuristics in low-validity environments (with just noise and no clear signals) simply because computers are more consistent.[1] Heuristics can outperform computers at tasks where the data points are muddled by noise. An intuitive heuristic approach is able to interpolate, extrapolate, and estimate. Thus, according to Gigerenzer, heuristics often outperform computers in making predictions.

General Use Heuristics

According to Gigerenzer, we have an adaptive toolbox containing an assortment of heuristics that we use according to the problem-solving task at hand. One heuristic is pattern recognition. According to psychologist James Reason,[7] when we see a pattern or an image, we first use a process called "similarity-matching." We ask, "Have I seen this before?" If not, we then use a process called "frequency-gambling." If we don't immediately recognize something, we will gamble that it is similar to something we have frequently seen in the past.

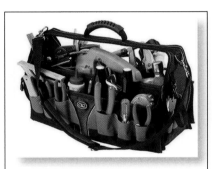

According to Gigerenzer, we have an adaptive toolbox of heuristics that we can use for various tasks.

Tools in the toolbox:
- *Pattern recognition*
- *Fast and frugal decision trees*
- *Tallying*
- *Default heuristic*
- *Trial and error*
- *Anchoring and adjusting*

We use the pattern-recognition heuristic to quickly diagnose life-threatening ventricular arrhythmias (Figure 5.2). Here, the heuristic enables us to treat the patient quickly, rather than going through rigorous data collection, which would cause harmful delay.

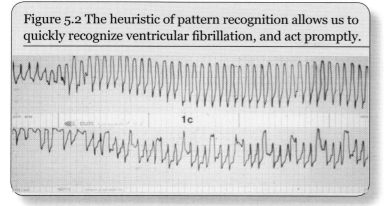

Figure 5.2 The heuristic of pattern recognition allows us to quickly recognize ventricular fibrillation, and act promptly.

Another heuristic is the simple branching algorithm (Figure 5.3). Gigerenzer has investigated how we use "fast and frugal" decision trees to quickly solve problems. To use this heuristic, we quickly sort through cues in a specific order; if we detect a highly valid cue, we stop searching for further cues.

An example of this heuristic is the use of the initial EKG in patients who present to the emergency room with chest pain. ST-segment elevation in 2 contiguous leads prompts a "STEMI alert" even before we have a complete history, physical exam, or laboratory data. ST-segment elevation, a highly valid cue, spurs a fast and frugal decision. The catheterization lab team is mobilized immediately, and the rest of the data are gathered later.

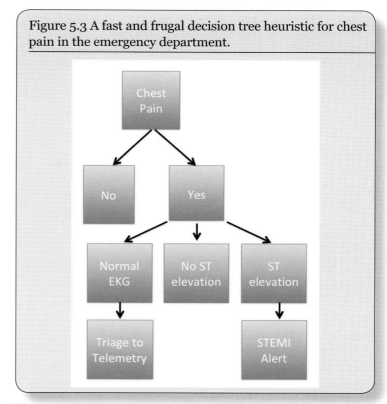

Figure 5.3 A fast and frugal decision tree heuristic for chest pain in the emergency department.

The initial EKG is also useful if it is normal. Years ago, I investigated how the initial EKG predicts complications of myocardial infarction. We observed that an initially normal or near-normal admission EKG was associated with a very low risk of in-hospital complications of an MI (Table 5.1).[8] Our study prompted hospitals to change their triage rules, sending these low-risk patients to a telemetry floor rather

Table 5.1 The Use of the Initial Electrocardiogram to Predict Complications of Acute Myocardial Infarction.[8]

	NEGATIVE ECG	POSITIVE ECG	
No life threatening complications	166	260	
Life threatening complications	1	42	
	167	302	469

Sensitivity=0.99, Specificity=0.14

LR(+)=TPR/FPR=sensitivity/1- specificity=1.15

LR(-)=FNR/TNR=1-sensitivity/ specificity=0.07

Sidebar 5.2 Benjamin Franklin on tallying (according to Gigerenzer[3]).

"My way is to divide half a sheet of paper by a line into two columns; writing over the one Pro, and over the other Con...I put down under the different heads short hints of the different motives that occur to me...and though the weight of reasons cannot be taken with precision of algebraic quantities, yet when each is thus considered... the whole matter lies before me... in what may be called moral or prudential algebra."

Benjamin Franklin in a letter to Joseph Priestly, 9/19/1772

than a coronary care unit. With a sensitivity of 0.99, a normal initial EKG has an excellent negative likelihood ratio of 0.07. A normal EKG in this setting has sufficiently high validity that it can be used in a fast and frugal decision algorithm.

Another frequently used heuristic in our toolbox is tallying. Simple tallying (i.e., adding up a series of unweighted cues) is an old tool whose merits Benjamin Franklin explained many years ago (Sidebar 5.2).[3]

A recent patient of mine, a 72-year-old woman who presented to the emergency department with chest pain, provides a useful example of tallying. The pros and cons for the diagnosis of unstable angina versus esophageal reflux are shown in Table 5.2. After the tallying, the pros and cons were fairly even. The tie went to the diagnosis of unstable angina, because of the

adverse consequences of missing the more serious diagnosis. Cardiac catheterization revealed critical stenoses in two vessels, and the patient responded well to coronary stenting.

Table 5.2 An example of the tallying heuristic. A 72 year old woman in the emergency department with chest pain.

PRO, UNSTABLE ANGINA	CON, REFLUX
History of CABG	History of reflux
Stent to a graft and protected left main 4 months ago	Patient thinks it's her reflux.
Diabetes, hyperlipidemia	Worse when lying down
Described as a pressure	Not exertional
Radiates to the axilla	Not relieved by nitroglycerin
Associated with shortness of breath	Persistent pain, yet normal EKG and cardiac enzymes

Psychologists Dawes and Corrigan have investigated the use of tallying.[9] They compared simple tallying with regression formulas and found that tallying was just as effective as the more complicated computer models. According to these investigators: "in most practical situations an un-weighted sum of a small number of 'big' variables will, on the average, be preferable to regression equations...The whole trick is to decide what variables to look at and then to know how to add." We use the tallying heuristic frequently in clinical medicine.

"Medical Heuristics"

Psychologists have shown us how we use general heuristics. Several processes in clinical medicine, taught to each generation of medical trainees, may be considered "medical heuristics" (Sidebar 5.3). Like general heuristics, they are learned mental processes that guide our decision making.

We are all trained to use a standardized history and physical. Systematic use of this process helps us get started and ensures completeness. Parts of the H&P, such as the review of systems, are simple checklists that force us to leave no stone unturned. Another medical heuristic is the narrative, which organizes clinical information so that we can use the pattern-recognition heuristic. By taking a complete history and physical, and then organizing the information into a narrative, we enable ourselves to see patterns that would otherwise be unrecognizable. We match a patient's narrative against "illness scripts," or prototypical disease narratives that we have stored away in memory.

Sidebar 5.3 "Medical heuristics"

- The standardized History and Physical

- The Narrative

- Early hypothesis generation

- Iterative hypothesis testing

- Problem-oriented medical record

- Use of the differential diagnosis

A good narrative, organized like any good story, is typically in chronological order. It is event-driven and detailed, and (most important) it has meaning. The narrative helps us organize cues so that we can make a connection between what we are observing and the underlying cause.

It is possible, though, to be fooled by a narrative. A fallacy called "post hoc, ergo propter hoc" (translated from the Latin as "after this, therefore because of this") describes how we can sometimes ascribe causality to events that occurred merely by coincidence. For example, the sun rises after the rooster crows in the morning, but it is obvious that the rooster crowing didn't cause the sun to rise.

The narrative can also lead to a fallacy, called confirmation bias, whereby we make selective use of facts to conform to a preconceived story. A good narrative can help us organize our thinking, but we should be careful to avoid these fallacies.

Another medical heuristic is early hypothesis generation. Studies by both Arthur Elstein[10] and Jerry Kassirer[11] showed that expert clinicians typically develop 3 to 5 hypotheses very early during the history-taking process. Through experience we learn to develop plausible conjectures about the patient's illness early in the process of obtaining a history. These early hypotheses facilitate a more targeted, proactive pursuit of the diagnosis. The line of questioning becomes more direct and less scattered. This approach requires good knowledge about manifestations of diseases, meticulous attention to the findings of a particular case, and the ability to make connections. It requires creativity, open-mindedness, and active thinking. In short, early hypothesis generation is a heuristic that turns a wild goose chase into a targeted, organized search for relevant cues.

Another medical heuristic is iterative hypothesis testing. This process allows the clinician to structure a problem and systematically work toward a logical conclusion by progressively redefining the problem statement. This heuristic requires suspended judgment. Although an expert clinician may jump to an early hypothesis, the savvy expert avoids leaping to an early conclusion. Iterative hypothesis testing helps us systematically avoid both hasty judgments and analysis paralysis.

Use of a problem list and a problem orientation is another medical heuristic. The problem list is a tool that helps us organize our thinking as we home in on a diagnosis. A patient may arrive in the emergency room reporting acute shortness of breath. After examining the patient and reviewing the chest X-ray, we formulate the problem statement as one of acute congestive heart failure. An echocardiogram is performed, showing an ejection fraction of 25%, and the problem is now redefined as acute systolic heart failure. Cardiac catheterization shows extensive triple-vessel coronary artery disease and evidence of prior myocardial infarcts. The diagnosis is refined further as acute systolic heart failure due to an ischemic dilated cardiomyopathy. Through iterative hypothesis testing and repeatedly updating a problem list, we can systematically work though a diagnostic problem-solving exercise.

Another medical heuristic is use of the differential diagnosis. By forcing ourselves to go through the mental process of asking "what else might this be?" we avoid jumping to conclusions and the fallacy of hasty generalization.

Strong diagnostic strategies rely on good information. Heuristics enable us to collect, sort, and organize cues so that they form a logical conclusion. Some cues are more valid than others. Some are strong, like the initial EKG in patients with chest pain. Others are weak, even misleading. Some cues, like Homan's sign for diagnosing deep venous thrombosis, are red herrings.

Likelihood Ratios to Measure the Validity of Cues

Chapter 4 discussed how likelihood ratios are useful for evaluating diagnostic tests. We can also use likelihood ratios to assess the strength of even small, everyday diagnostic cues. Use of likelihood ratios is well summarized in an excellent book, *The Rational Clinical Examination: Evidence-based Clinical Diagnosis* by Simel and Rennie.[12]

Figure 5.4 shows the positive likelihood ratios for various diagnostic cues for acute myocardial infarction. The likelihood ratios are the true-positive rate divided by the false-positive rate, plotted on an ROC curve. The black curve shows the ROC curve for a moderate test. Cues that are plotted above and to the left of the black curve are reasonably valid. For patients with suspected myocardial infarction, radiation to the left arm is not a very strong cue, but radiation to both arms is much stronger. Several other cues are also shown in the figure.

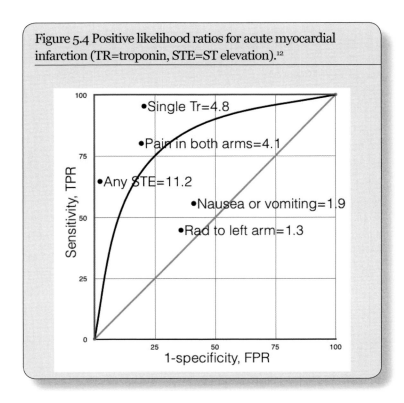

Figure 5.4 Positive likelihood ratios for acute myocardial infarction (TR=troponin, STE=ST elevation).[12]

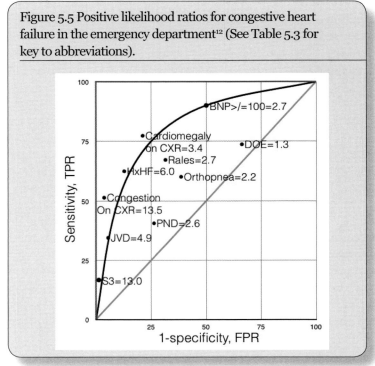

Figure 5.5 Positive likelihood ratios for congestive heart failure in the emergency department[12] (See Table 5.3 for key to abbreviations).

Figure 5.5 shows positive likelihood ratios for a variety of cues that could be used to diagnose congestive heart failure in the emergency room. As shown, an s3 gallop has a very high positive likelihood ratio. An s3 gallop also has very high specificity. If it's there, the patient almost certainly has congestive heart failure. If it's absent, however, this cue isn't very helpful. The sensitivity is too low.

A BNP (brain natriuretic peptide) level, in contrast, is quite sensitive. If it is negative, the probability of congestive heart failure is very low. This test is less specific, however, with frequent false positives. The positive and negative likelihood ratios of various cues for congestive heart failure are shown in Table 5.3.

Table 5.4 lists positive and negative likelihood ratios for cues for a variety of noncardiac disorders. As noted previously, some likelihood ratios are asymmetric. For some, the positive finding may be much stronger (palpation of AAA >3.0 cm, for example), whereas for others the negative finding may be much stronger (such as d-dimer for pulmonary embolism).

Heuristics enable us to collect and sort cues. Knowing the strength of cues helps us plug in the most appropriate heuristic. A particularly strong cue may lead to a fast and frugal decision-tree heuristic. A series of moderate cues may lead to the tallying heuristic. Likelihood ratios can help us gauge the validity of the cues that influence our decisions. Knowing the likelihood ratios for common clinical findings can help us calibrate our intuition.

Table 5.3 Likelihood ratios for findings of congestive heart failure.[12]

FINDING	LR(+)	LR(-)
Congestion on Chest X-Ray (CXR)	13.5	0.48
S3 gallop	13.0	0.83
History of Congestive Heart Failure (HxHF)	6.0	0.45
Jugular Venous Distention (JVD)	4.9	0.65
Cardiomegaly on Chest X-ray	3.4	0.33
BNP(brain natriuretic peptide) ≥ 100	2.7	0.1
Rales on exam	2.7	0.41
Paroxysmal Nocturnal Dyspnea (PND)	2.6	0.7
Orthopnea	2.2	0.65
Dyspnea on Exertion (DOE)	1.3	0.48

Table 5.4 Likelihood ratios for common clinical findings for various diagnoses.[12]

DISORDER	LR(+)	LR(−)
Palpation of abdominal aortic aneurysm (AAA) >3.0 cm	12	0.72
Bruit for diagnosing carotid stenoses >70% in symptomatic patients	1.6	0.6
Abdomino-jugular reflex	4.4	0.5
Murphy's sign for cholecystitis	2.8	0.5
D-dimer for Deep Venous Thrombosis	2.1	0.19
D-dimer for Pulmonary Embolus	1.7	0.09
Pulse deficit for aortic dissection	5.7	0.7
Diastolic murmur for aortic dissection	1.4	0.9
Wide mediastinum for aortic dissection	2.0	0.3

Heuristics, when well calibrated and used properly, can help us develop strong diagnostic strategies that more reliably lead to the correct diagnosis. Strong diagnostic strategies use reliable data and emphasize strong cues. Strong strategies are targeted and logical. Although our decisions are largely intuitive, they can be supported by computers for searching, organizing, remembering, and reminding. The emergence of the electronic medical record, based on logical problem lists, holds much promise in this regard. Finally, strong diagnostic strategies are supported by metacognition (thinking about how we think) and by analytical thinking, to double-check our work. We can use heuristics more effectively if we consciously monitor how we employ them.

Strong diagnostic strategies:

• Use reliable, objective, unambiguous data (strong cues).

• Are targeted, prospective, active.

• Have a logical order.

• Use skilled intuition (careful use of heuristics and accurate estimates of personal probability).

• Are aided by computers (searching, organizing, remembering, and reminding).

• Are supported by analytical thinking (double checks, causal reasoning, meta cognition).

In thinking about the simplifying effects of heuristics, I am reminded of a story that my father (an engineer) told me years ago. A tractor-trailer was too tall for the Lincoln Tunnel and became jammed in the tunnel entrance. The authorities called in engineers, from nearby universities, who arrived with their slide rulers and expert knowledge. The experts were arguing about the best course of action when a boy rode up on his bicycle and asked, "Why don't you just let the air out of the tires?" Sure enough, the simple solution worked and the problem was solved. In medicine, things can get very complicated. Heuristics can offer elegant simplicity that can make us more effective.

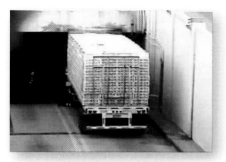

A tractor trailer truck stuck in the Lincoln Tunnel.

Herbert Simon summarizes how we use heuristics to process cues: "The situation has provided a cue; this cue has given the expert access to information stored in memory, and the information provides the answer. Intuition is nothing more and nothing less than recognition."[13] Experts learn with experience how to use intuition, cues, and heuristics. If we understand how heuristics work and if we recognize their pros and cons, we can use them effectively in practice.

References:

1. Kahneman D, Klein G. Conditions for intuitive expertise: A failure to disagree. The American Psychologist. 2009; 64: 515-526

2. Kahneman D. Thinking, Fast and Slow. New York: Farrar, Straus and Giroux; 2011.

3. Gigerenzer G, Todd PM, and the ABC Research Group. Simple Heuristics That Make Us Smart. New York, Oxford University Press, Inc. 1999.

4. Pólya G. How to solve it; a new aspect of mathematical method. Princeton, N.J.: Princeton University Press; 1971.

5. Simon H. Invariants of human behavior. Annual Review of Psychology. 1990; 41:1-20

6. Simon HS. Models of My Life. New York. Harper Collins Publishers; 1991.

7. Reason J. Human Error. New York, NY, Cambridge University Press; 1990.

8. Brush JE, Jr., Brand DA, Acampora D, Chalmer B, Wackers FJ. Use of the initial electrocardiogram to predict in-hospital complications of acute myocardial infarction. The New England Journal of Medicine. 1985; 312:1137-1141

9. Dawes RM, Corrigan, B. Linear models in decision making. Psychological Bulletin. 1974; 81 (2):95-106

10. Elstein AS, Shulman, L.Sl, Sprafka, S.A. Medical Problem Solving: An Analysis of Clinical Reasoning. Cambridge, MA: Harvard University Press; 1978.

11. Kassirer JP, Gorry, G.A. Clinical problem solving: A behavioral analysis. Ann Intern Med. 1978; 89:245-255

12. Simel DL, Rennie D, Keitz SA. The rational clinical examination: Evidence-based clinical diagnosis. New York: McGraw-Hill; 2009.

13. Simon H. What is an explanation of behavior? Psychological Science 1992; 3(3):150-160

Chapter 6

Therapeutic Decision Making

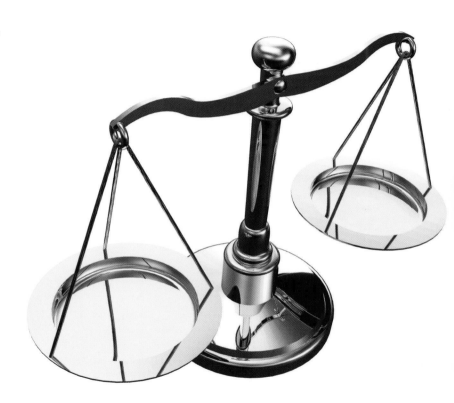

Therapeutic decision making is a choice between gambles —
an exercise in weighing options. It starts with defining the
options using estimates of probability. In the end, the goal is
to choose the option that gives the patient the best chance of
a favorable outcome.

Therapeutic decisions can be distorted if we are not careful. Consider the following example. A pharmaceutical sales rep comes to your office bringing lunch. He shows you a graphic (Figure 6.1) that says dronedarone reduced the primary endpoint in the ATHENA trial by 24%, with an impressive P value of <0.0001. You come away satisfied that this drug looks good. (You may not realize it, but you also feel an unconscious sense of obligation to the sales rep for the lunch.)

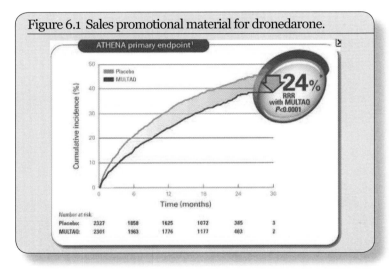

Figure 6.1 Sales promotional material for dronedarone.

Nevertheless, you decide to check this claim by consulting the New England Journal of Medicine paper.[1] There you find that the primary endpoint — first hospitalization due to a cardiovascular event, or death — occurred in 31.9% of the treatment group and 39.4% of the placebo group. That represents a 19% relative reduction (apparently, the 24%

figure was initially reported at a national meeting but is not reflected in the published data). The difference between the randomized groups was mainly due to the reduction in the rate of hospitalizations. A 7.5% absolute risk reduction for the combined endpoint is starting to look less impressive.

The inverse of this absolute risk reduction, the number needed to treat (NNT), is 13. The drug was discontinued because of adverse events in 12.7% of the treatment group and 8.1% of the placebo group, yielding a number needed to harm (at least enough to discontinue the drug) of 22. The average follow-up was 21 months, and the drug costs $276 per month.

You think to yourself, "I would need to treat 13 patients for an average of 21 months, at a total cost of more than $75,000, to prevent one hospitalization due to a cardiovascular event or one death. If I treat an additional 9 patients, I would cause enough harm to cause one patient to discontinue the drug." Hmmm, not so good after all.

This example shows the power of marketing and how our therapeutic decision making can be distorted by relying on relative risk reduction, which exaggerates the findings of a study. Absolute risk reduction and NNT more accurately represent the effects of a drug or intervention.

The goal of therapeutic decision making is to improve the outcome for a patient through some type of intervention. We use the results of randomized controlled trials to guide treatment decisions because we believe that a particular treatment strategy will yield better outcomes, on average, than a different strategy would (Figure 6.2). The difference between the intervention and some alternative is best described in absolute terms. Our dronedarone example shows how relative improvement tends to exaggerate the treatment effect.

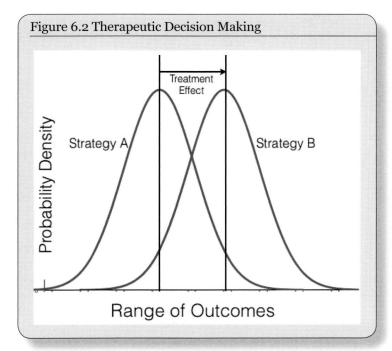

Figure 6.2 Therapeutic Decision Making

Some treatments, like antibiotics for community-acquired pneumonia or urinary tract infection, have a dramatic and consistent treatment effect. As shown in Figure 6.3, almost all treated patients get much better.

For most cardiovascular treatments, however, the numerical effect is often less dramatic. In many drug trials, the absolute risk reduction may be only a couple of percentage points (Figure 6.4). Nonetheless, if the primary endpoint is mortality, even a small absolute risk reduction would be important. Many trials of cardiovascular drugs use a combined endpoint — usually death, nonfatal myocardial infarction, or stroke — to increase the trial's efficiency. The trials are often mega-trials, enrolling thousands of patients in the hope of showing a statistically significant effect that may actually be small in absolute terms.

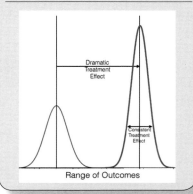

Figure 6.3 Treatment effect for highly effective treatments such as antibiotics for community acquired pneumonia or urinary tract infection.

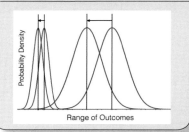

Figure 6.4 The absolute treatment effect for typical drugs for cardiovascular disease, shown on the left, may be only a few percentage points.

83

Figure 6.5 shows the promotional sales material for clopidogrel, based on the CURE trial,[2] boasting an impressive 20% relative reduction in the combined endpoint. Careful scrutiny, however, reveals that the absolute risk reduction is a less impressive 2.1%.

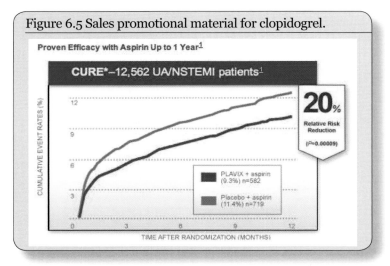

Figure 6.5 Sales promotional material for clopidogrel.

The absolute risk reduction in a clinical trial is an average risk reduction. Not every patient responds the same way. As shown in Figure 6.6, most drugs have a heterogeneity of treatment effects. Clopidogrel, for example, is a prodrug, and genetic variability can affect how well the drug is converted to its active form. Also, evidence shows that clopidogrel has interactions with other drugs that could affect patients who are taking the other drugs. Another example is warfarin, which has many drug interactions that can cause heterogeneity

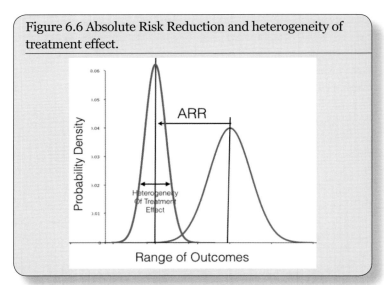

Figure 6.6 Absolute Risk Reduction and heterogeneity of treatment effect.

in the treatment effect. Variation in age, gender, or patient adherence can also cause treatment-effect heterogeneity. Most trials report the effect of the treatment in subgroups, to identify those that may have received more or less benefit from the drug. However, the statistics of subgroup analysis can be misleading; therefore, subgroup analysis should be considered hypothesis-generating rather than a basis for a firm conclusion.

Statistical tests for interaction can help determine whether there is an independent effect of a treatment in a particular subgroup. For example, in several trials comparing bypass surgery with percutaneous coronary intervention, there is an interaction between the type of revascularization and diabetes. In these trials comparing revascularization strategies, the subgroup of patients with diabetes tend to do better with coronary artery bypass surgery than with percutaneous coronary intervention.

Many drugs are double-edged swords. The decision to use these drugs requires careful analysis of the potential efficacy as well as the potential for serious side effects, such as bleeding complications. In this regard, the treatment decision becomes an arbitrage where we bet that the increase in efficacy will be numerically greater and clinically more important than the increase in risk (Figure 6.7). For treatments that are double-edged swords, such as fibrinolytic therapy, antiplatelet agents, or anticoagulants, it is important to consider the magnitude of potential benefit and potential risk to determine the net clinical benefit. Different subgroups, such as elderly patients, may have different degrees of benefit and risk. Prasugrel, for example, is an effective treatment for acute coronary syndrome, but it may confer a higher risk for hemorrhagic stroke in elderly patients and in patients with a history of stroke.[3]

Patients may have strong preferences and unique perceptions about side effects. A patient with a strong fear of having a stroke, for example, may prefer a particular treatment option, even if it carries a higher risk for death, to avoid the stroke risk. A thorough, frank discussion with each patient is needed to determine his or her preferences and to ensure that we are choosing the treatment option that maximizes efficacy while avoiding potential side effects, especially those to which a particular patient has a strong aversion (Figure 6.8).

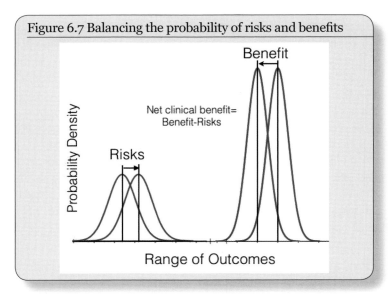

Figure 6.7 Balancing the probability of risks and benefits

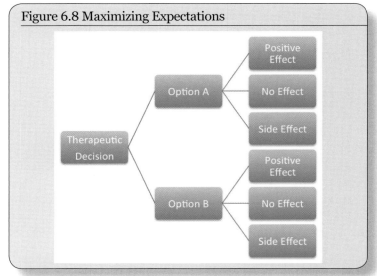

Figure 6.8 Maximizing Expectations

Number Needed to Treat

As noted, absolute risk reduction is better than relative risk reduction in representing the efficacy of a drug, device, or treatment strategy. The inverse of the absolute risk reduction, the number needed to treat (NNT), may be even more intuitive. The relationship between absolute risk reduction and NNT is shown in Figure 6.9. Use of NNT was proposed in 1988 by Andreas Laupacis and colleagues at McMaster University.[4]

How does NNT work? Consider a trial of a drug showing an absolute risk reduction of 7%. This means that 7 events are avoided per 100 patients treated. The reciprocal of this relationship tells us that there would be 100 patients treated per 7 events avoided. By dividing 100 by 7, we can say that there would be 14 patients treated per one event avoided. Thus, the number needed to treat is 14. The NNT is the number of patients that we need to treat to avoid one event — so, the smaller the better. As a rule of thumb, an NNT less than 50 is satisfactory, corresponding to an absolute risk reduction of at least 2%. The NNT should be should be less than one half, but preferably less than one fourth, the number needed to harm. The relationship among baseline risk, relative risk reduction, and NNT is shown in Table 6.1. For conditions with a very low baseline risk, the NNT becomes very large for even a modest relative risk reduction. In effect, it is hard to make a low-risk patient better.

For conditions with a high baseline risk, the NNT becomes very small. Let's take an extreme example. For a skydiver, the baseline risk of dying without a parachute is 100%. The NNT for the strategy of using a parachute is 1.

The effectiveness of prevention therapy is critically dependent on the baseline risk of the outcome that we intend to prevent. For example, patients with persistent atrial fibrillation can benefit from chronic anticoagulation therapy, but if the baseline risk of thromboembolism in a particular patient is low, the absolute risk reduction may be small and NNT may be very high. Various factors can increase the risk of thromboembolism in patients with atrial fibrillation and we can use simple tools such as the CHADS2 score or available

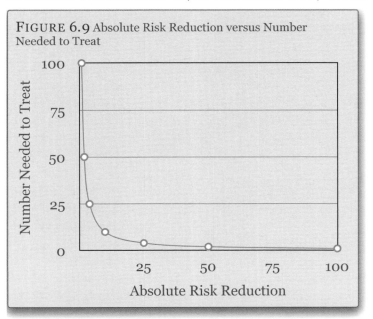

FIGURE 6.9 Absolute Risk Reduction versus Number Needed to Treat

hand-held applications to estimate the baseline risk.[16] Another example is the primary prevention of atherosclerotic cardiovascular disease. Treatment with statin drugs has been shown to reduce the risk of dying or having a heart attack or stroke. Recent guidelines have recommended using a risk calculator to estimate the 10 year risk of a cardiovascular event and making treatment decisions based on the estimate of baseline risk.[17]

NNT is a useful, intuitive tool for comparing the efficacy of various treatment strategies. The NNTs for common cardiovascular treatments are shown in Table 6.2. Using NNT, we can summarize a study in a single declarative sentence. For example, the BHAT trial showed that you need to treat 34 patients with acute myocardial infarction with a beta-blocker for 25 months to prevent one death.[7] The SAVE trial showed that you need to treat 20 patients with congestive heart failure and an ejection fraction ≤40% with an ACE inhibitor for 42 months to prevent one death.[8] In these trials, the NNTs are low, given the powerful treatment effect of the tested drugs — so powerful that the two treatments have become performance measures. Consistently using those treatments has been designated as a marker of good-quality medicine. Not treating patients with AMI and CHF, respectively, with each of these drugs would be a mistake.

Number needed to treat is a very personal notion of the probability of a treatment effect. Imagine bringing 20 untreated patients with congestive heart failure and an ejection fraction of ≤40% into a room and saying, "If I start all of you on an ACE inhibitor, over the next 42 months I will save the life of one of you."

Therapeutic decision making for our patients is a choice between gambles that requires knowledge and skill. The

Table 6.1 Effect of baseline risk and relative risk reduction on the number needed to treat. (Adapted from Laupacis, et al.[4])

BASE-LINE RISK	Relative Risk Reduction						
	50	40	30	25	20	15	10
	Number Needed to Treat						
0.9	2	3	4	4	6	7	11
0.6	3	4	6	7	8	11	17
0.3	7	8	11	13	17	22	33
0.2	10	13	17	20	25	33	50
0.1	20	25	33	40	50	67	100
0.05	40	50	67	80	100	133	200
0.01	200	250	333	400	500	667	1000
0.005	400	500	667	800	1000	1333	2000
0.001	2000	2500	3333	4000	5000	6667	10000

Table 6.2 Number needed to treat (NNT) for many common cardiovascular drugs and interventions.

INTER-VENTION	TRIAL	GROUP	TIME	EVENT RATES	NNT
Aspirin	Meta-analysis[5]	AMI	24 months	12.8 vs 5.5	14
Heparin	Theroux[6]	Unstable angina	6 days	10.4 vs 7.9	40
Clopidogrel	CURE[2]	ACS	9 months	11.4 vs 9.3	48
Beta Blockers	BHAT[7]	AMI	25 months	10 vs 13	34
ACEI (Captopril)	SAVE[8]	EF≤40%	42 months	20 vs 25	20
ARB (valsartan)	Val-HeFT[9]	EF≤40%	23 months	29 vs 32	30
Hydralazine/ nitrates	V-HeFT[10]	HF	3 years	36 vs 47	10
Bidil	A-HeFT[11]	AA HF	20 months	6.2 vs 10.2	25
Simvastatin	4S[12]	CAD	5.4 years	8 vs 12	25
AICD	SCD-Heft[13]	EF≤35%	45.5 months	22 vs 29	14
Warfarin	Meta-analysis[14]	Afib	1 year	2.4 vs 4.5	48
TAVR	Partner[15]	AS	1 year	31 vs 51	5

knowledge about a treatment strategy can be captured in a short statement using the number needed to treat, which distills what we need to carry in our working memory. NNT can make therapeutic decisions more intuitive. NNT and number needed to harm can help us understand the net clinical benefit for various treatment options. Combining knowledge of therapeutic efficacy with knowledge of the preferences and values of individual patients is key to making the best therapeutic decisions for our patients.

Therapeutic decisions are based on evidence from clinical research. In the next chapter, we will discuss how to evaluate clinical research and how to incorporate evidence into our thinking.

References:

1. Hohnloser, SH, et al. For the ATHENA Investigators. Effect of dronedarone on cardiovascular events in atrial fibrillation. N Engl J Med 2009; 360:669=8-678

2. The CURE Trial Investigators. Effects of clopidogrel in addition to aspirin in patients with acute coronary syndromes without ST-segment elevation. N Engl J Med 2001; 345:494-502

3. Wiviott SD, et al. Prasugrel versus clopidogrel in patients with acute coronary syndromes. N Engl J Med 2007; 357:2001-2015

4. Laupacis A, Sackett DL, Roberts RS. An assessment of clinically useful measures of the consequences of treatment. The N Engl J Med 1988; 318:1728-1733

5. Antithrombotic Trialists' Collaboration. Collaborative meta-analysis of randomised trials of antiplatelet therapy for prevention of death, myocardial infarction, and stroke in high risk patients. BMJ 2002; 324:71

6. Theroux P, et al. Aspirin, heparin, or both to treat acute unstable angina. N Engl J Med 1988; 319:1105-11

7. A randomized trial of propranolol in patients with acute myocardial infarction. I. Mortality results. JAMA 1982 26:247(12);1707-14

8. Pfeffer MA, et al. Effect of captopril on mortality and morbidity in patients with left ventricular dysfunction after myocardial infarction - Results of the survival and ventricular enlargement trial. N Engl J Med 1992; 327:669-677.

9. Cohn JN, et al. A randomized trial of the angiotensin-receptor blocker valsartan in chronic heart failure. N Engl J Med 2001; 345:1667-1675

10. Cohn JN, et al. A comparison of enalapril with hydralazine-isorsorbide dinitrate in the treatment of chronic congestive heart failure. N Engl J Med 1991; 325:303-10

11. Taylor AL, et al. Combination of isosorbide dinitrate and hydralazine in blacks with heart failure. N Engl J Med 2004; 351:2049-57

12. The Scandinavian Simvastatin Survival Study Group. Randomized trial of cholesterol lowering in 4444 patients with coronary heart disease: The Scandinavian Simvastatin survival study (4S). Lancet 1994; 344:1383-89

13. Bardy GH, et al. Amiodarone or an implantable cardioverter-defibrillator for congestive heart failure. N Engl J Med 2005; 352:225-37

14. Van Walraven, et al. Oral anticoagulants versus aspirin in nonvalvular atrial fibrillation: An individual patient meta-analysis. JAMA 2002; 288(19);2441-2448.

15. Smith CR, et al. For the PARTNER Trial Investigators. Transcatheter versus surgical aortic-valve replacement in high-risk patients. N Engl J

16. January CT, Wann LS, Alpert JS, Calkins H, Cigarroa JE, Cleveland JC Jr, Conti JB, Ellinor PT, Ezekowitz MD, Field ME, Murray KT, Sacco RL, Stevenson WG, Tchou PJ, Tracy CM, Yancy CW. 2014 AHA/ACC/HRS guideline for the management of patients with atrial fibrillation: a report of the American College of Cardiology/American Heart Association TaskForce on Practice Guidelines and the Heart Rhythm Society. J Am Coll Cardiol 2014; 64:e1–76

17. Goff DC Jr, Lloyd-Jones DM, Bennett G, Coady S, D'Agostino RB Sr, Gibbons R, Greenland P, Lackland DT, Levy D, O'Donnell CJ, Robinson JG, Schwartz JS, Shero ST, Smith SC Jr, Sorlie P, Stone NJ, Wilson PWF. 2013 ACC/AHA guideline on the assessment of cardiovascular risk: a report of the American College of Cardiology/American Heart Association Task Force on Practice Guidelines. J Am Coll Cardiol 2014; 63:2935–59

Chapter 7

Evidence-based Medicine

"Evidence-based medicine is the conscientious, explicit, and judicious use of current best evidence in making decisions about the care of individual patients...

...Good doctors use both individual clinical expertise and the best available external evidence, and neither alone is enough."

-David Sackett[1]

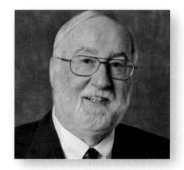

David L. Sackett, McMaster University. One of the founders of evidence-based medicine.

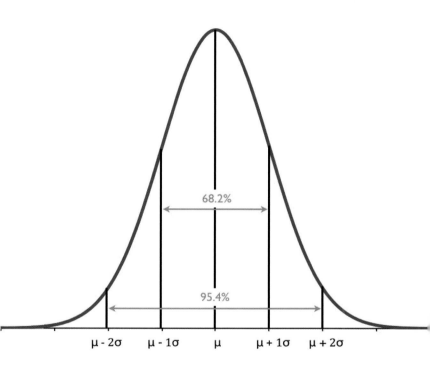

Science is a quantitative discipline; it uses numbers to measure, analyze, and explain nature. Evidence-based medicine tells us how to practice by the numbers, how to use objective scientific data to guide medical decisions. We have already discussed how numbers can calibrate our intuitive decisions, such as using likelihood ratios as we make judgments about diagnostic testing and even physical exam findings. We discussed using the number needed to treat to calibrate therapeutic decision making. But how can we intuitively incorporate new knowledge and research into our practices? How should new evidence, as we judge its importance, shift our thinking? For this, we again rely on probability and Bayesian logic. We often fall back on the anchoring and adjusting heuristic, properly calibrated, to judge the clinical significance of new scientific evidence.

To apply evidence-based medicine, we have to think like both a player and a manager. A player's focus is to watch the ball; a manager thinks about winning the most games during a season. With evidence-based medicine, we must focus on each patient and each opportunity without losing sight of the bigger picture. We want to achieve the best possible outcomes for the most patients over the long run.

Brief Review of Statistics

To use evidence-based medicine, we have to know something about statistics. We will briefly review some basic statistics that we can use to analyze new evidence, to help us decide whether new scientific evidence should change how we practice.

Mark Twain wasn't very enamored of statistics. While it is possible to lie with statistics, it is also nearly impossible to demonstrate scientific truth without statistics. The use of statistics is crucial for interpreting results from clinical trials.

Statistics don't give us the truth. They help us make inferences about the truth by supplying a method for accepting or rejecting new evidence. Twain was right to be skeptical, even

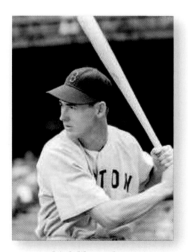

Think like a player.
Focus on each patient.

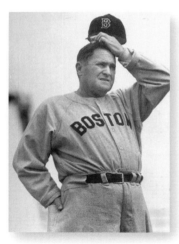

Think like a manager.
Play the percentages.

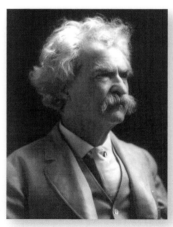

Mark Twain: "There are three
types of lies. There are lies,
damn lies, and statistics."

cynical. There are sometimes reasons to doubt the statistical results of clinical trials. Some of these problems are listed in Sidebar 7.1. Strong economic forces are at work when clinical trials are reported. A clinical trial could have a billion-dollar impact on a medical products company. Investigators may have economic entanglements and conflicts of interest. Furthermore, the results of any research are likely to affect investigators' careers and reputations. The vast majority of companies and investigators do honest research, but it pays to be a little skeptical.

Sidebar 7.1 Caveat emptor. There are many reasons to be a savvy consumer of the medical literature.

Industry-sponsored trials

Investigator bias, conflict of interest

Publication bias

Data manipulation (Vioxx)

Lack of access to patient-level data

Ghostwritten articles

Seeding trials

Industry funding for CME

Direct-to-consumer advertising

Statistics can be descriptive or inferential. Descriptive statistics are like batting averages. They are simple counts. We can count mortality rates, the number of patients with congestive heart failure readmitted within 30 days, or the number of patients with acute myocardial infarction getting aspirin at discharge. With descriptive statistics, the numbers speak for themselves and require little interpretation.

Inferential statistics require some interpretation. They allow us to form a conjecture about a population, using a sample of that population. With inferential statistics, we use probability to assess whether our inference about a population is valid. The larger the sample, the more the sample looks like the

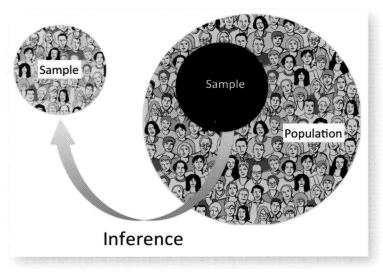

Inferential statistics. We make a statistical inference about a population by analyzing a sample.

93

entire population, making the statistical inference about the population more valid.

Inferential statistics is a form of induction. Statistics help us make predictions on the basis of past observations, by putting numbers on the likelihood of the predictions and on the validity of the observations. However, we must be careful about our interpretations. As David Hume noted long ago, there is no guarantee that the future will conform to the past. Statistics can sometimes lead us to wrong conclusions.

Statistics use probability to make inferences about samples and populations. Central limit theorem, mentioned in Chapter 3, provides the basis for much of statistical thinking. According to this theorem, a large sample, properly drawn, resembles the population from which it is drawn (Figure 7.1). From parameters like the mean and the standard deviation of a sample, we can make inferences about the larger population. Alternatively, if we know parameters about a larger population, we can draw inferences about whether some group is a sample from that population. In addition, if we know something about two samples, we

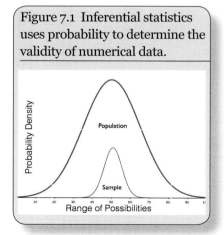

Figure 7.1 Inferential statistics uses probability to determine the validity of numerical data.

can infer whether the samples are from the same population or from different populations.

Inferential statistics enable us to make correlations, examine differences, or make estimates, as shown in Figure 7.2. We can use statistics to evaluate categorical variables or continuous variables. An example of a categorical variable is mortality: Each patient is unequivocally categorized as either dead or alive. For categorical variables, we express the presence or absence of events as rates, and we can use logistic regression to analyze correlation and tests such as chi-square analysis to analyze differences.

We can also use statistics to evaluate continuous variables, such as serum cholesterol level or blood pressure. A continuous variable is expressed as a mean and a standard deviation

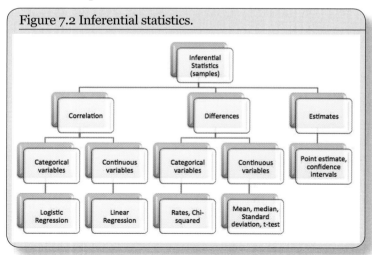

Figure 7.2 Inferential statistics.

from the mean. For continuous variables, we can use linear regression to analyze correlation and tests such as the t-test to analyze differences.

For estimates, we can calculate confidence intervals to express the precision of a point estimate. Confidence intervals are discussed later in this chapter.

Types of Clinical Studies

We use statistics to evaluate the validity of clinical trials. Randomized controlled trials are generally considered to provide the most compelling evidence, since the randomization process eliminates most sources of bias.

A randomized controlled trial must be carefully planned, to ensure that it is properly conducted. Such trials are expensive, and a lot is riding on the results. As shown in Table 7.1, there are four possible outcomes for the validity of a clinical trial. Investigators design a trial to avoid either a false-positive result, called a Type I error, or a false-negative result, called a Type II error. Generally, the investigators set the risk of a Type I error, called the alpha level, at 0.05, and the risk of a Type II error, called the beta level, at 0.20. The power of the trial is a measure of the trial design's ability to avoid a false-negative result. The power of a trial is 1 minus the beta level.

Standard computer programs help investigators pinpoint the number of patients required in each treatment group to detect a specified amount of difference in outcomes among the treatment groups, given a prespecified alpha and beta level. In

some ways, a clinical trial resembles an investigation of a patient with a diagnostic test. Both use a test to determine the true state of nature, and both have four possible outcomes for how well the true state of nature and the test results match up (Table 7.2).

Other types of trials are used when randomization is impossible. It would be unethical to test the effect of smoking by randomizing young people to cigarettes or a placebo, for example, so we use observational cohort studies, such as the Framingham Heart Study, to address such questions. In

Table 7.1 Structure of a RCT

	TRUE STATE OF NATURE	
	Drug A is better than Comparator	Drug A is no better than Comparator
+Trial	Correct TP Power=1-β	Type I error FP Risk of error=α
-Trial	Type II error FN Risk of error= β	Correct TN

Table 7.2 Similar to the Structure of a Diagnostic Test

	TRUE STATE OF THE PATIENT	
	+ Disease	- Disease
+Test	TP	FP
-Test	FN	TN

observational cohort studies, data are collected prospectively to ensure that they are complete and adequately address the investigative questions.

Another type of study, the case-control study, uses retrospective comparisons of a disease group with a non-diseased group to look at exposure rates to various factors that might be the cause of the disease. This type of study yields odds ratios, which measure the association between a disease and different factors that might be causing it. Finally, there are physiologic studies that add to our understanding of disease and can guide our decision making.

Multiple clinical trials can be combined in a meta-analysis to give us a single estimate of a treatment effect. By combining the weighted results of multiple trials, a meta-analysis may show an effect that was not apparent in any of the trials alone. Problems arise because negative trials are underreported, which can bias a meta-analysis toward a positive treatment effect.

Investigators frequently report subgroup analyses of clinical trials. A trial design may include an analysis of prespecified subgroups, but generally a trial is not planned or sized to draw firm conclusions about subgroups. With subgroup analysis, there is a risk that chance findings will appear to show statistical significance. Subgroup analyses should be considered hypothesis-generating, providing the basis for further research, rather than conclusive.

Some of the terms that are commonly used in clinical research are listed in Sidebar 7.2.

Sidebar 7.2 Some terms used in clinical trials.

Risk, or event rates - proportion of events in each of the treatment arms. It is the number of subjects with an event in a group divided by the total number of subjects in that group (either the treatment group or the control group).

Relative Risk, or risk ratio (RR) - risk of the event in the treatment group/risk of the event in the control group.

Relative Risk Reduction (RRR) - absolute risk reduction/risk of the event in the control group.

Absolute risk reduction (ARR) - difference in event rates between treatment group and control group.

Odds - the number of subjects with an event divided by the number of subjects without an event in either the treatment group or the control group.

Odds Ratio (OR) - the odds of an event occurring in the treatment group divided by the odds of an event occurring in the control group. Odds and risk are different, therefore, the OR is different from the RR. The OR is always further from the point of no effect (where OR=1 and RR=1) than the RR. If the treatment group has a higher event rate than the control group, the OR will be larger than the RR. If the treatment group has a lower event rate than the control group, the OR will be smaller than the RR. At low values (<0.1), odds and risk are almost equal, therefore, the OR is almost equal to the RR when events are rare.

Hazard ratio - broadly equivalent to relative risk. In clinical trials using survival data, it uses data collected at different times.

Statistical Significance and the P-Value

When we use statistics to show a difference between two groups, the standard method is to start by assuming that there is no difference between the two groups — the so-called "null hypothesis." For a clinical trial, the null hypothesis is the proposition that the treatment under investigation has no effect. The statistical analysis of a trial yields a P value, which is often misunderstood to represent the probability that the null hypothesis is true. This incorrect interpretation of the P value overestimates the probability of the null hypothesis.[2] The correct interpretation of a P value is the probability of deriving the data, or a more extreme data set, given the assumption that the null hypothesis is true.

Imagine a clinical trial, comparing treatments A and B, that is repeated many times (Figure 7.3). If there is no difference between A and B (i.e., the null hypothesis is true), most of the repeated trials would in fact show no difference and would pile up in the center of the probability density curve, as shown in Figure 7.3. By chance, however, some of the repeated trials would show that A is slightly better and others that B is slightly better. In the figure, the further we move on the x-axis from the center, the greater the difference between treatment A and treatment B, and the less likely that a trial would show such a difference. We can place a point on the graph, the prespecified alpha level, beyond which a larger difference between A and B would be very unlikely. If one trial showed a larger difference between A and B than the difference specified by the alpha level, we would say that a very improbable event occurred, given

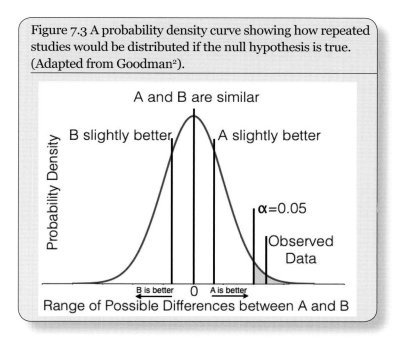

Figure 7.3 A probability density curve showing how repeated studies would be distributed if the null hypothesis is true. (Adapted from Goodman[2]).

that we didn't anticipate a difference between A and B. The observed data from such a trial would line up at the extreme end of the probability density curve, as shown.

When a trial is designed, the alpha level is usually set at 0.05. If the P value of the observed data is less than 0.05, one can conclude that a very improbable event occurred (assuming the null hypothesis is true). Given the preset alpha level and the observed data, we can conclude that the chance of observing that data set, given that the null hypothesis is true, is less than 1 in 20. The observed data may be so improbable that we could reasonably question whether the null hypothesis is true, and we could conclude that the null hypothesis should be rejected. To calculate the true probability of the null hypothesis, we have to use some Bayesian logic.[3] First, we estimate the prior probability of the null hypothesis. The estimated prior probability might be based on prior trials, personal observations, or theoretical considerations. Having set a prior probability, we can use the strength of the new evidence to calculate the posterior probability of the null hypothesis.

The relationship between the prior probability and the posterior probability of the null hypothesis is shown in Table 7.3. The first column shows a variety of P values and their associated z-scores (which is the trial's observed effect divided by the standard error of the observed data). The second column shows the strength of the evidence, expressed by a minimum Bayes factor, which is a likelihood ratio. It is the likelihood of the observed data, given the null hypothesis, divided by the likelihood of the observed data, given the best alternative hypothesis. The minimum Bayes factor is discussed further in Appendix 3.

We can multiply the Bayes factor by the prior odds of the null hypothesis to yield the posterior odds of the null hypothesis. A range of prior probabilities and the corresponding posterior probabilities are shown in the third and fourth columns.

The calculation of the probability of the null hypothesis is similar to the Bayesian process we used, in chapter 4 to calculate posttest probability using likelihood ratios of diagnostic tests.

We convert probability to odds (odds = p/[1 − p]). We then multiply the prior odds by the minimum Bayes factor. Finally, we convert the posterior odds back to probability (p = odds/[1 + odds]) to yield the posterior probability of the null hypothesis. For example, the second row in Table 7.3 shows that the Bayes factor for a clinical trial with a P value of 0.05 is 0.15. If we are initially indifferent about the trial, our prior probability of the null hypothesis might be 0.5, making the prior odds = 1. Multiplying 0.15 by 1 yields a posterior odds of 0.15. We turn the posterior odds of 0.15 back to probability: 0.15/(1 + 0.15) = 0.13. Thus, a clinical trial with a P value of 0.05 would change our prior probability of the null hypothesis from 0.5 to 0.13. The P value fallacy would lead us to believe that the probability that the null hypothesis is true is 0.05, but when we incorporate our prior convictions about the trial and do the calculation, we find that the probability that the null hypothesis is true is higher: 0.13.

The nomogram in Figure 7.4 helps us visualize how we can use the anchoring and adjusting heuristic and Bayesian logic to decide whether to accept the results of a clinical trial. Here, the evidence (the Bayes factor) is fixed, but the prior probability of the null hypothesis varies, depending on whether we are initially neutral, a skeptic, or a believer. If we are initially skeptical, our initial probability of the null hypothesis is very high. Let's take an extreme example: a hypothetical research study showing that pigs fly. Of course, our initial conviction is that pigs don't fly, so we would reject the results of the clinical trial, no matter what the P value was.

Table 7.3 Relation between p values, minimum Bayes factors and probability of the null hypothesis. (From Goodman[3])

P VALUE (Z SCORE)	MINIMUM BAYES FACTOR	CHANGE IN THE NULL HYPOTHESIS		STRENGTH OF EVIDENCE
		From	To no less than	
0.10 (1.64)	0.26 (1/3.8)	75	44	Weak
		50	21	
		17	5	
0.05 (1.96)	0.15 (1/6.8)	75	31	Moderate
		50	13	
		26	5	
0.03 (2.17)	0.095 (1/11)	75	22	Moderate
		50	9	
		33	5	
0.01 (2.58)	0.036 (1/28)	75	10	Moderate to strong
		50	3.5	
		60	5	
0.001 (3.28)	0.005 (1/216)	75	1	Strong to very strong
		50	0.5	
		92	5	

On the other hand, a clinical trial may evaluate a drug that we view as very promising. We may start out as a believer, and a positive trial result will reinforce our prior conviction that the null hypothesis is unlikely. Figure 7.4 shows that, depending on our prior convictions about a study, our posterior probability of the null hypothesis will vary greatly.

Critics say that this method for determining the probability of the null hypothesis is too subjective because it requires an arbitrary

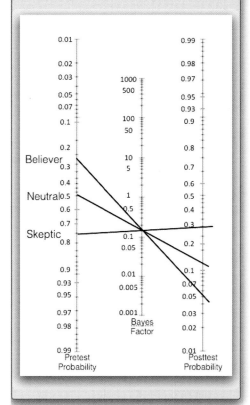

FIGURE 7.4 Nomogram showing how we can use anchoring and adjusting to determine the posterior probability of the null hypothesis, depending on whether we start out neutral, as a believer, or as a skeptic.

estimate of the prior probability of the null hypothesis. To counter this argument, we can use a range of prior probabilities to calculate a range of corresponding posterior probabilities, as shown in Table 7.3. By using this Bayesian approach, we can avoid being oversold on new evidence. Jumping to conclusions about a clinical trial when the findings are just not plausible would be a form of base-rate neglect. It would be a mistake to disregard our prior convictions about the probability of the null hypothesis and accept a P<0.05 at face value.

Take the TACT randomized trial, which showed that disodium EDTA chelation therapy reduced the risk for adverse cardiovascular outcomes among patients with prior myocardial infarction.[4] Chelation therapy has questionable biologic rationale, so one might be fairly skeptical about its true effectiveness. Let's say that we are 75% sure that this treatment is ineffective — that is, 75% sure that the null hypothesis is true. Given a prior probability of 75% that the null hypothesis is true, a trial with a P value of 0.036 (z = 2.1) would give us a posterior probability of about 25% that the null hypothesis is true.

If you think a conclusion from a trial has a 1 in 4 chance of being wrong, it is not a good idea to let the trial results change how you treat your patients. I don't doubt that the trial was properly performed and the data are correct, but a P value is calculated using methods based on probability. Whether you are tossing coins, pulling random balls from an urn, or performing a randomized controlled trial, occasionally improbable things will happen.

Confidence Intervals

Another problem with the P value is that although it gives a measure of the evidence, it does not characterize the magnitude of an observed treatment effect in a trial.[2] A trial with a small effect but a large sample size can have the same P value as a trial with a large effect and a small sample size. Investigators have tried to overcome this problem by using confidence intervals (Figure 7.5). A recent paper by Kaul and Diamond explains how to do this.[5] The estimate of relative treatment effect and the confidence intervals around the relative treatment effect can be displayed to show whether the trial results are both statistically significant and clinically important. To use this method, we have to establish a minimal clinically important difference (MCID) between the two comparison groups in the trial.

As shown in Figure 7.5, you may decide ahead of time that a 15% relative reduction in the primary endpoint is necessary to convince you that a new treatment is clinically important. The first trial in Figure 7.5 shows results that are statistically insignificant and clinically unimportant. The second trial has a confidence interval that meets the threshold for clinical importance but also crosses the line of identity for statistical significance. Take the Theroux trial evaluating heparin for patients with unstable angina.[17] The trial was small, not quite reaching statistical significance at the 0.05 level, yet the trial has been deemed clinically important and has broadly affected clinical practice. The third example is a trial that is statistically significant but may not be clinically important, like a 2002 meta-analysis of trials of GP IIb/IIIa antagonists.[20] This

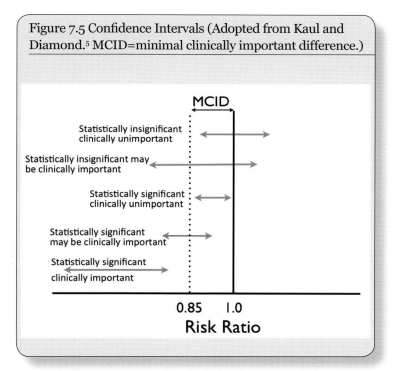

Figure 7.5 Confidence Intervals (Adopted from Kaul and Diamond.[5] MCID=minimal clinically important difference.)

huge analysis yielded a significant P value, but the absolute difference in the combined endpoint between the treatment group and the control group was only 1.3%. The NNT was 77. Next, we have trials that are statistically significant and may be clinically important, such as the CURE trial, whose combined endpoint had an NNT of 48.[18] Finally, numerous trials are both statistically significant and clinically important, such as GISSI, BHAT, SAVE, CONSENSUS, or RALES. Many of these trials are listed in Table 7.4.

Number Needed to Treat

As shown in Table 7.4, the number needed to treat gives us a single number that helps us understand the clinical significance of a trial. As mentioned in chapter 6, the NNT can be put into a simple declarative sentence that concisely summarizes the trial. For example, the CONSENSUS trial showed that you need to treat 7 patients with class III or IV systolic heart failure with enalapril for one year to prevent one death. This single statement — with the trial name, the magnitude of the treatment effect, the entry criteria, the drug, the duration of study, and the outcome measure — makes it easy to grasp the clinical importance of the study.

Cleland and colleagues examined the treatment effects of multiple heart failure drugs and showed that for patients with class III or IV heart failure, the cumulative effects of ACE inhibitors, beta-blockers, and aldosterone antagonists can have an even greater effect.[24] The NNT for this combination is only 3!

Non-inferiority Trials

Several published trials compare newer anticoagulants with warfarin for patients with nonvalvular atrial fibrillation. These "noninferiority trials" do not aim to show that a new treatment is superior to another, but instead use statistical methods to analyze whether the new treatment is not inferior to an existing one. Noninferiority trials are used to evaluate a new drug or device when comparison with placebo would be unethical because the existing treatment has proven efficacy. A new

Table 7.4 NNT for common cardiovascular treatments.

TREATMENT	NNT	ENDPOINT	TRIAL
ACEI, Class 3,4 HF	7	Mortality	Consensus[6]
Spironolactone Class 3,4 HF	9	Mortality	Rales[7]
Hydralazine/ nitrate	10	Combined	V-HeFT[8]
Aspirin	14	Combined	Trialists[9]
AICD	14	Mortality	SCD-HeFT[10]
B blocker HF	18	Mortality	Copernicus[11]
ACEI	20	Mortality	SAVE[12]
Bidil	25	Combined	A-HeFT[13]
Simvasttin	25	Mortality	4S[14]
ARB	30	Combined	Val-HeFT[15]
B blocker MI	34	Combined	BHAT[16]
Heparin	40	Combined	Theroux[17]
Clopidogrel	48	Combined	CURE[18]
Warfarin	48	Combined	Meta-analysis[19]
GPIIb/IIIa	77	Combined	Meta-analysis[20]

treatment, however, may have ancillary advantages over an existing treatment, such as safety, tolerability, convenience, or cost. The trial design requires making assumptions about the margin of decreased efficacy that one would consider acceptable before considering replacing a proven existing treatment with the new treatment. It is important for the trial designer to make these assumptions before conducting the trial, to avoid gerrymandering the margin of decreased efficacy after the fact. Noninferiority trials require a larger sample size than standard randomized controlled trials do. Noninferiority trials can also show superiority, and it is valid to infer superiority from a noninferiority trial. However, RCTs that are initially designed as superiority trials cannot be changed to a noninferiority trial after the fact, again to avoid post-hoc gerrymandering to achieve a positive result. Table 7.5 shows results from three recent noninferiority trials of anticoagulant medications. In both the RE-LY trial and the ARISTOTLE trial, the study drug was significant for noninferiority as well as for superiority, compared with warfarin.

Table 7.5 Examples of recent non-inferiority trials.

DRUG	TRIAL	# OF PATIENTS	RESULTS
Dibigatran (a direct thrombin inhibitor)	RE-LY[21]	18,113	1.11% vs. 1.69% (p<0.001 for NI, p<0.001 for superiority)
Rivaroxaban (a Factor Xa inhibitor)	ROCKET-AF[22]	14,264	1.7% vs. 2.2% (p<0.001 for NI)
Apixaban (a Factor Xa inhibitor)	ARISTOTLE[23]	18,201	1.25% vs. 1.6% (p=0.01 for superiority

Trial Endpoints

To evaluate the importance of any clinical trial, we must consider the endpoint that is tested. To increase trial efficiency, many clinical trials use a combined endpoint. By combining endpoints, investigators can reduce the number of patients that they have to enroll for the trial to show a statistically significant difference. Combined endpoints, however, can create problems for interpretation. An endpoint may be the combination of death and myocardial infarction, for example, and death is obviously a much more serious endpoint than a laboratory elevation of cardiac enzymes. Nevertheless, the endpoints are lumped together. When interpreting the study, we should assess which endpoints are driving the overall study result.

Some trials use surrogate endpoints, which are laboratory results or findings that presumably predict that the study drug has some other effect on an important outcome. In many trials, however, surrogate endpoints create problems, as shown in Sidebar 7.3. The CAST study sought to decrease premature ventricular contractions after myocardial infarction and unexpectedly caused an increase in mortality.[25] Lowering HDL cholesterol with torceptrapib ran into similar problems.[26] The AIM-High trial showed that treating hyperlipidemia with niacin resulted in a higher stroke rate in treated patients.[27] Trials that are designed to reduce a surrogate endpoint should be viewed

Sidebar 7.3 Problems with Surrogate Endpoints

Cardiac Arrhythmia Suppression Trial (CAST) evaluating encainide and flecainide[24]

Surrogate:PVCs after MI

Study drugs increased mortality.

Torceptrapib trial[25]

Surrogate: HDL

Study drug increased mortality.

AIM-High trial of niacin[26]

Surrogate: HDL

Study drug increased CVA rate.

with caution and should not influence practice patterns as much as trials that directly analyze actual patient outcomes.

Also, most trials are not sized to detect a small increase in the rate of serious complications. If a study drug causes liver failure, it is usually obvious and the trial would be halted prematurely. Cardiac side effects, however, can hide in the data because cardiac conditions are common. It wasn't obvious initially, but post-market research by tenacious investigators revealed an increase in cardiac complications secondary to use of Vioxx and Avandia.[28,29]

One has to maintain a healthy degree of skepticism before accepting the results of a clinical trial and incorporating them into practice (Sidebar 7.4). Large trials may achieve statistical significance, but the practitioner must assess the clinical significance of the findings. Ideally, the NNT for an intervention should be <50, and much less than the number needed to harm. The cost of the treatment is also a consideration. The practitioner has to consider how generalizable the study results are to the population he or she is treating. Finally, the practitioner has to ask whether there are any significant biases or conflicts of interest that may have distorted the results of the trial.

Many issues cannot be evaluated in clinical trials. To examine these issues, we can use observational studies. Outcomes research gives us a glimpse of what is happening in the real world, compared with the relatively artificial world defined by the entry criteria of a clinical trial. Outcomes research can examine a range of issues related to safety, timeliness of care,

---

Sidebar 7.4 Healthy Skepticism about Clinical Trials

Large trials: statistical significance, BUT clinical significance?

NNT<50, substantial endpoint, number needed to harm >>NNT. Cost? Duration of study?

Combined endpoints

Primary vs. secondary endpoints

Surrogate endpoints

Subgroup analysis

Generalizability

Industry sponsorship

Author conflicts of interest

---

efficacy, efficiency, and patient preferences. These studies offer valuable feedback on how we are really doing in practice and can shift our thinking about it. Outcomes research has revealed lapses in care and has led to quality improvement initiatives. According to Yale researcher Harlan Krumholz, the goal of outcomes research is "to increase the likelihood that patients achieve the outcomes they desire through better information, better decisions, and better health care delivery."[30]

The philosopher William James once wrote, "There can be no difference anywhere that doesn't make a difference elsewhere."[31] This has become the maxim of pragmatic philosophy and could be the motto of outcomes research. Medical care, with its basic science, clinical research, systems of care, and medical reasoning, ultimately has to make a difference. The goal of medical care is to make sick people better and to make well people less likely to get sick. The ultimate measure of success is how well we do that in the real world.

Outcomes research uses observational data rather than experimental data. Thus, outcomes studies are more prone to bias than controlled clinical trials, and the results can sometimes be misleading.[32] Outcomes research sometimes creates more questions than answers, but it can generate important hypotheses and may confirm that medical care is making a real difference in the uncontrolled environment of the real world with real people.

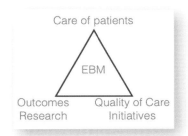

Outcomes research gives us feedback on how we care for patients in the real world. (EBM-evidence-based medicine)

Outcomes research has entered a new era with the Patient-Centered Outcomes Research Institute (PCORI), established in 2010 by the Patient Protection and Affordable Care Act. PCORI's mission is "to support the production of well-validated scientific evidence to assist the nation in making informed decisions about a broad range of health care-related issues."[33]

Outcomes research examines medical care from a patient's perspective. It helps us develop a basis for shared decision making, which is key for quality improvement. Quality improvement is the subject of the next chapter.

References:

1. Sackett DL, et al. Evidence-based medicine: what it is and what is isn't. BMJ 1996; 312:71

2. Goodman SN. Toward evidence-based medical statistics. 1: the p value fallacy. Ann Intern Med 1999; 130(12): 995-1004.

3. Goodman SN. Toward evidence-based medical statistics. 2: The Bayes Factor. Ann Intern Med 1999;130(12): 1005-1013

4. Lamas GA, et al. Effect of disodium EDTA chelation regimen on cardiovascular events in patients with previous myocardial infarction: The TACT randomized trial. JAMA 2013; 309(12):1241-1250

5. Kaul S, Diamond GA. Trial and Error: How to avoid commonly encountered limitations of published clinical trials. J Am Coll Cardiol 2010; 55(5):415-27

6. The Consensus Trial Study Group. Effects of enalapril on mortality in severe congestive heart failure. Results of the cooperative North Scandinavian Enalapril Survival Study (CONSENSUS). N Engl J Med 1987; 316:1429-35

7. Pitt B, et al. The effect of spironolactone on morbidity and mortality in patients with severe heart failure. N Engl J Med 1999; 341:709-17.

8. Cohn JN, et al. A randomized trial of the angiotensin-receptor blocker valsartan in chronic heart failure. N Engl J Med 2001; 345:1667-1675.

9. Antithrombotic Trialists' Collaboration. Collaborative meta-analysis of randomised trials of antiplatelet therapy for prevention of death, myocardial infarction, and stroke in high risk patients. BMJ 2002; 324:71.

10. Bardy GH, et al. Amiodarone or an implantable cardioverter-defibrillator for congestive heart failure. N Engl J Med 2005; 352:225-37.

11. Packer M, et al. Effect of carvedilol on survival in severe chronic heart failure. N Eng J Med 2001; 344:1651-58.

12. Pfeffer MA, et al. Effect of captopril on mortality and morbidity in patients with left ventricular dysfunction after myocardial infarction - Results of the survival and ventricular enlargement trial. N Engl J Med 1992; 327:669-677.

13. Taylor AL, et al. Combination of isosorbide dinitrate and hydralazine in blacks with heart failure. N Engl J Med 2004; 351:2049-57.

14. The Scandinavian Simvastatin Survival Study Group. Randomized trial of cholesterol lowering in 4444 patients with coronary heart disease: The Scandinavian Simvastatin survival study (4S). Lancet 1994; 344:1383-89.

15. Cohn JN, et al. A randomized trial of the angiotensin-receptor blocker valsartan in chronic heart failure. N Engl J Med 2001; 345:1667-1675.

16. A randomized trial of propranolol in patients with acute myocardial infarction. I. Mortality results. JAMA 1982 26:247(12);1707-14.

17. Theroux P, et al. Aspirin, heparin, or both to treat acute unstable angina. N Engl J Med 1988; 319:1105-11

18. The CURE Trial Investigators. Effects of clopidogrel in addition to aspirin in patients with acute coronary syndromes without ST-segment elevation. N Engl J Med 2001; 345:494-502.

19. Van Walraven, et al. Oral anticoagulants vs aspirin in nonvalvular atrial fibrillation: An individual patient meta-analysis. JAMA 2002;288(19);2441-2448.

20. Boersma E, Harrington RA, Moliterno DJ, et al. Platelet glycoprotein IIb/IIIa inhibitors in acute coronary syndromes: a meta-analysis of all major randomized clinical trials. Lancet 2002;359:189-98.

21. Connolly SJ, et al. Dibigatran versus warfarin in patients with atrial fibrillation. N Eng J Med 2009; 361:1139-1151.

22. Patel MR, et al. Rixaroxaban versus warfarin in nonvalvular atrial fibrillation. N Engl J Med 2011; 365:883-91.

23. Granger CB, et al. Apixaban versus warfarin in patients with atrial fibrillation. N Eng J Med 2011; 365:981-92.

24. Cleland JGF, Clark AL. Delivering the cumulative benefits of triple therapy to improve outcomes in heart failure: Too many cooks will spoil the broth. J Am Coll Cardiol 2003;42(7):1234-1237.

25. Echt DS et al. Mortality and morbidity in patients receiving encainide, flecainide, or placebo - the Cardiac Arrhythmia Suppression Trial. N Engl J Med 1991; 324:781-8.

26. Barter PJ, et al. Effects of torcetrapib in patients at high risk for coronary events. N Eng J Med 2007; 357:2109-22.

27. The AIM-HIGH Investigators. Niacin in patients with low HDL cholesterol levels receiving intensive statin therapy. N Engl J Med 2011; 365:2255-67.

28. Mukherjee D, et al. Risk of cardiovascular events associated with selective COX-2 inhibitors. JAMA 2001;286(8):954-9.

29. Nissen SE and Wolski K. Effect of rosiglitazone on the risk of myocardial infarction and death from cardiovascular causes. N Engl J Med 2007; 356:2457-71.

30. Krumholz HM. Real-world imperative of outcomes research. JAMA 2011;306(7):754-755.

31. Haack S, Lane R. Pragmatism old & new : Selected writings. Amherst, NY: Prometheus Books; 2006.

32. Ioannidis JP. Why most published research findings are false. PLoS medicine. 2005;2:e124

33. Clancy C, Collins FS. Patient-Centered Outcomes Research Institute: The intersection of science and health care. Sci Transl Med 2010;37(2):37.

Chapter 8

Improving the Quality of Care

"Simply put, health care quality is getting the right care to the right patient at the right time — every time."

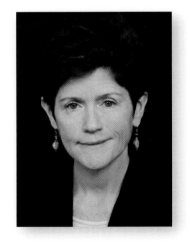

- Carolyn Clancy, Director, Agency for Healthcare Research and Quality. Statement before the Subcommittee on Health Care, Committee on Finance, U.S. Senate, March 18, 2009

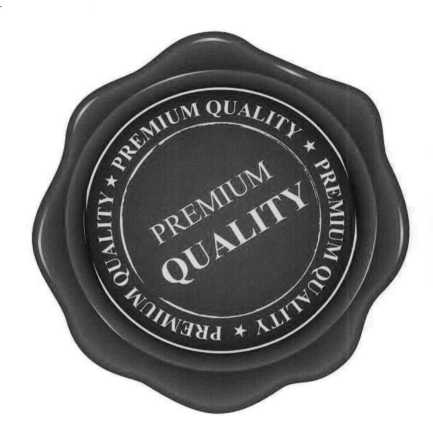

Getting the right care to the right patient at the right time every time requires good judgment. In previous chapters we discussed the internal thought processes that lead to good judgment. We discussed how critical thinking, recalibration, and reflection can improve decision making. In this chapter we will discuss external factors, such as organizational structure and process of care, that affect decisions and outcomes. We will explore how quality is defined, performance is measured, and systems are redesigned to improve quality. The goal of quality-of-care efforts is to produce healthcare that is measurably better, less variable, and more reliable (Figure 8.1).

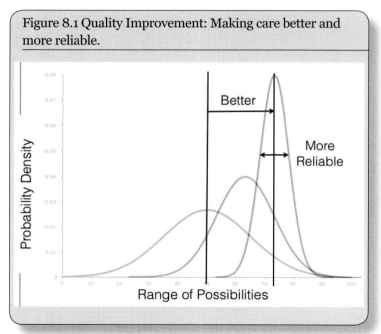

Figure 8.1 Quality Improvement: Making care better and more reliable.

For the past two decades, quality of care has become a major focus of payers, regulators, professional organizations, academics, patient-advocacy groups, and others. Thought leaders and researchers have worked to explicitly define quality and have developed methods to measure it. The field has developed into a discrete subspecialty, with its own specialized terminology, taxonomies, measurement tools, experts, conferences, and journals. Many people and organizations are now working to improve patient care. Public reporting, pay-for-performance programs, and awareness campaigns have engaged the public and practicing physicians in learning more about quality of care.

Consumers want the highest-quality product for the lowest cost. Our customers — patients, families, and purchasers — are demanding greater value. The internet now offers abundant information for comparison shopping, and patients are becoming savvier about using indicators of quality to choose their care.

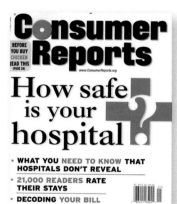

The Institute of Medicine (IOM), a division of the National Academy of Sciences, galvanized public attention on healthcare quality by publishing two influential books in 1999 and 2001. The first, *To Err is Human: Building a Safer Health System*, revealed the problem of medical errors.[1] It garnered considerable public attention by revealing the estimate that tens of thousands of patients die each year as a result of medical errors. The second book, *Crossing the Quality Chasm: A New Health System for the 21st Century*, focused more on the gap between the medical care that patients should receive and the care they do receive.[2] Both books outlined various remedies that employ system redesign and methods adapted from industry to improve quality.

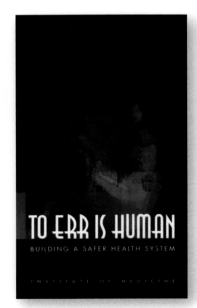
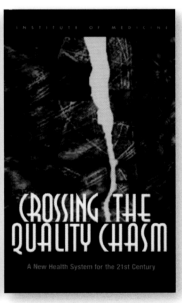

Published by the Institute of Medicine in 1999.

Published by the Institute of Medicine in 2001

Defining Quality of Care

The IOM authors define quality as "the degree to which health services for individuals and populations increase the likelihood of desired health outcomes and are consistent with current professional knowledge."[2] A simpler definition of quality might be "meeting expectations."

The most fundamental definition of quality relates to patient safety. The physician's dictum for centuries has been *primum non nocere*, or "first do no harm." Avoiding harm, such as medication errors, hospital-acquired infections, falls, and other accidents, has become a high priority for hospitals.

The authors of *Crossing the Quality Chasm* defined high-quality healthcare as 1) safe, 2) effective, 3) patient-centered, 4) timely, 5) efficient, and 6) equitable. Providing effective care means reliably delivering care that is based on scientific evidence. Being patient-centered means "providing care that is respectful of and responsive to individual patient preferences, needs, and values and ensuring that patient values guide all clinical decisions." Equitable care "does not vary in quality because of

Healthcare should be:

• Safe

• Effective

• Patient-centered

• Efficient

• Timely

• Equitable

personal characteristics such as gender, ethnicity, geographic location, and socioeconomic status."

From a physician perspective, quality is often defined as 1) complying with evidenced-based medicine, or "doing the right thing," and 2) procedural quality, or "doing the right thing right." The "right thing" is largely determined through the consensus opinion of medical experts. To create quality standards, professional organizations have developed expert consensus documents that list guideline recommendations and performance measures for specific diseases and procedures, and appropriate use criteria for diagnostic tests and interventions. Failure to do the right thing might be either an overuse error (when potential harm exceeds the potential benefit) or an underuse error (when an appropriate test or therapy is not used).

Failure to do the right thing right is called a misuse error. To track how well we perform, several professional organizations have developed clinical data registries that provide a mechanism for accurately monitoring performance.

Avendis Donabedian, a visionary in the quality field, defined two elements of physician performance: one related to technical performance (using knowledge, judgment, and skill) and another related to interpersonal relationships (the ability to communicate, modify care according to individual preferences, and engage the patient in fruitful collaboration).[3]

To define standards of care, many professional organizations have produced clinical practice guidelines. These expert

---

What is Quality?

Safety
> "First do no harm."

> Avoiding falls, medication and transfusion errors, infections.

Evidence-based medicine
> "Doing the right thing"

> Avoiding underuse and overuse errors.

> Focus of guidelines, performance measures, and appropriate use criteria

Procedural performance
> "Doing the right thing right"

> Avoiding misuse errors.

---

consensus documents address the growing complexity of science and promote adherence to evidence-based medicine. The IOM defines clinical practice guidelines as "systematically developed statements to assist practitioner and patient decisions about appropriate health care for specific clinical circumstances." The American Academy of Pediatrics developed the first guideline more than 50 years ago. Since then, almost every medical organization has produced its own set of guidelines. The Agency for Healthcare Research and Quality maintains www.guidelines.gov, which links to more than 900 guidelines.

The American College of Cardiology and the American Heart Association have collaborated to produce 18 current clinical practice guidelines, all developed using a rigorous and consistently methodical approach. In these guidelines, each recommendation is classified according to its strength, as shown in Figure 8.2. Class I and III recommendations are assigned to procedures or treatments that clearly should or should not be done. They are the do's and the don'ts. Class II recommendations, assigned to procedures where there is conflicting or incomplete evidence, are the grey areas that require reasoning and intuitive judgment. As noted in Chapter 1, about 64% of the ACC/AHA guideline recommendations fall into this category.[4] Along with a classification number, each recommendation is assigned a level of evidence, based on the strength of the available evidence that support the recommendation. Practitioners can calibrate their thinking about procedures by referring to guideline recommendations, which are based on the consensus of nationally recognized experts.

Figure 8.2 Classification of recommendations and levels of evidence in ACC/AHA guidelines.

Class I

Benefit >>> Risk

Procedure/ Treatment **SHOULD** be performed/ administered

Class IIa

Benefit >> Risk
Additional studies with focused objectives needed

IT IS REASONABLE to perform procedure/ administer treatment

Class IIb

Benefit ≥ Risk
Additional studies with broad objectives needed; Additional registry data would be helpful

Procedure/Treatment **MAY BE CONSIDERED**

Class III

Risk ≥ Benefit
No additional studies needed

Procedure/Treatment should **NOT** be performed/administered **SINCE IT IS NOT HELPFUL AND MAY BE HARMFUL**

Level A: Recommendation based on evidence from multiple randomized trials or meta-analyses
Multiple (3-5) population risk strata evaluated; General consistency of direction and magnitude of effect

Level B: Recommendation based on evidence from a single randomized trial or non-randomized studies
Limited (2-3) population risk strata evaluated

Level C: Recommendation based on expert opinion, case studies, or standard-of-care limited (1-2) population risk strata evaluated

Very

Guidelines create clinical standards and have the potential to reduce unjustified variation. From guidelines we can develop other quality-improvement tools, such as standard order sets, critical pathways, and discharge checklists.

For many diagnostic procedures, particularly imaging procedures, research is lacking and evidence is insufficient to underpin firm guideline recommendations about proper use. It is difficult to design a research study to examine how an imaging test affects long-term outcomes, and there are few randomized controlled trials of diagnostic tests. A new type of expert consensus document, called appropriate use criteria (AUC), offers guidance about these procedures.[5] The goal of AUC guidelines is to reduce overuse errors and to maximize the value of diagnostic testing and procedures.

Measuring Quality of Care

Measuring quality of care is not easy. Avendis Donabedian had this thoughtful reflection on measuring quality: "An apparatus of formal assessment is necessary to assure fairness, predictability, stability, and legitimacy. Nothing is more destructive to morale than a procedure for assessment based on unverified impressions, using private criteria, that is fitfully and selectively applied."[3]

To measure the performance of hospitals and clinics, Donabedian defined three dimensions of quality: structure, process, and outcome. A structure measure describes the attributes of the setting in which care is delivered, such as characteristics of the facility, the qualifications of the providers, nursing ratios, administrative support, and so on. Process measures capture how well we apply diagnostic tests and therapies; these elements of care are the actionable drivers of outcome. In other words, process measures are actions, identified by clinical research, which front line clinicians can

Donabedian's
Dimensions of Quality:

1. Structure-attributes of the care setting.

2. Process-use of tests and therapies.

3. Outcome-measurable changes of healthcare status.

Good structure leads to good process, which leads to good outcomes.

do to influence patient outcomes. Outcome measures are the results, or the measurable changes in the healthcare status of an individual or population, such as mortality, morbidity, symptomatic status, and cost. According to Donabedian, good structure leads to good process, which leads to good outcomes.

Performance can be tracked using clinical data registries, which are used to collect key clinical data prospectively. In a registry, data elements are defined and standardized to ensure consistent data collection, thereby allowing hospitals to compare their current performance with their past performance and with that of similar hospitals. The data in these registries are collected specifically for quality improvement, unlike insurance claims data, which are collected for billing purposes. Claims data are widely available but lack the detail necessary for precisely measuring clinical activity. Clinical data registries are better for quality measurement, but collecting data for them requires additional labor and expense. These registries can facilitate accurate measurement of procedural outcomes.

Outcome measures are often risk-adjusted. Without risk adjustment, an outcome measure could encourage a practitioner to cherry-pick cases and avoid high-risk patients. Risk adjustment can level the playing field so that similar institutions can be compared. A risk-adjustment model includes variables that independently predict some outcome, such as mortality.

Using a large, robust database, investigators first perform a univariate analysis to test potential predictive variables that might plausibly predict the outcome in question. Next, multivariate logistic regression is used to test candidate variables and then define a set of variables that have independent predictive value and statistical significance. The analysis gives the odds ratios for predictive variables, showing the strength of the association between the predictive variable and the outcome that is being predicted. The resulting model can be used to predict an outcome variable from the weighted sum of the predictive variables.

A risk-adjustment model can be used to calculate an expected outcome, such as the mortality rate for an institution, adjusted for case mix. From this, an observed to expected ratio (O:E ratio) can be calculated. For an outcome such as mortality, an O:E ratio of 1 means that the institution performed as expected, greater than 1 means that the observed mortality was higher than expected and less than 1 means that the institution did better than expected.

Risk-adjustment models are not perfect. A model can over-fit the data, perfectly conforming to past performance but poorly

predicting future performance because of noisy data. Also, unmeasured variables may confound the risk adjustment. Nevertheless, use of risk-adjusted outcomes measures is increasing. Outcomes measures are the ones that make the most sense to patients, and there is a growing public outcry for more transparency on outcomes.

The Centers for Medicare and Medicaid Services has worked with other agencies, including the Joint Commission, to define performance measures for hospital performance. CMS reports hospital performance through its website, hospitalcompare. hhs.org, which features a variety of process measures and risk-adjusted outcomes measures for disease conditions. A sample screenshot from that website is shown in Figure 8.3. Other agencies and patient-advocacy groups are creating their own definitions of quality of care, and many are now publicly

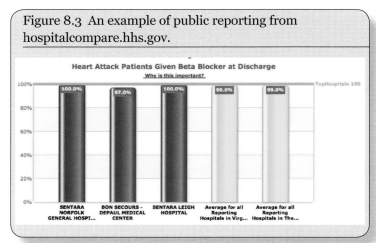

Figure 8.3 An example of public reporting from hospitalcompare.hhs.gov.

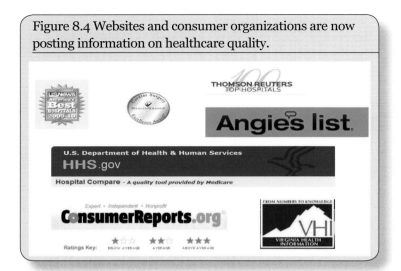

Figure 8.4 Websites and consumer organizations are now posting information on healthcare quality.

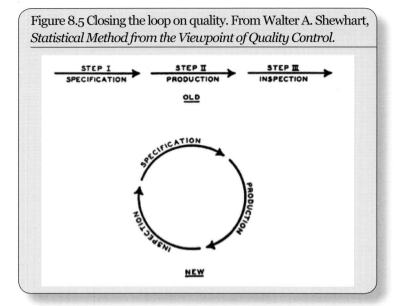

Figure 8.5 Closing the loop on quality. From Walter A. Shewhart, *Statistical Method from the Viewpoint of Quality Control*.

reporting the results online. A few examples are shown in Figure 8.4.

Improving Quality of Care

Many national organizations have initiated efforts to improve the quality of care. Donald Berwick, former CEO of the Institute for Healthcare Improvement and a CMS administrator, has been a leader in quality improvement. He and others have suggested that we apply quality-improvement methods from other industries to healthcare.[6] For example, we can learn from the manufacturing industry and from engineers like Walter Shewhart and W. Edwards Deming.

Figure 8.5, from a 1939 book by Walter Shewhart,[7] shows an old method of production that is open-ended and a new method that closes the loop on quality. Shewhart's newer method of quality control specifies a quality standard, designs a production method to meet that quality standard, and uses inspection to close the loop. If inspection shows that quality is not "up to spec," the production process is changed to ensure that the product meets the specifications. This approach is quite applicable to medicine because our published guidelines and performance measures explicitly define the quality standards and provide us with the necessary specifications.

James Reason, a cognitive psychologist who has studied how human factors affect industrial quality, described three types of common errors in his book *Human Error*.[8] One, frequently seen in medicine, is a skill-based slip. This error results from inattention, distraction, or preoccupation. Imagine the following scenario: "While I was discharging Mr. Smith, I was interrupted by a page and was called urgently to the emergency room. Because of that, I failed to discharge Mr. Smith on a beta-blocker after his recent myocardial infarction. It just slipped my mind."

The second type of error, a rule-based mistake, involves misapplying a rule. Imagine this example: "I didn't start Mrs. Jones on an ACE inhibitor for her congestive heart failure because her creatinine was slightly elevated and I thought ACE inhibitors were contraindicated in patients with elevated creatinine." Here, the ACE inhibitor should have been started because of a mortality benefit and the creatinine should have been followed. Most likely, the creatinine would have remained stable, and the patient would have benefitted from the ACE inhibitor.

The third type of error, a knowledge-based error, reflects a basic misunderstanding of the rules of evidence-based medicine, such as "I didn't know that patients with myocardial infarction benefit from beta-blockers."

My own observation is that most of our errors are skill-based slips related to distraction, fatigue, and time pressure.

Reminders, checklists, decision aids, and hard-stops in the electronic medical record can help limit this type of error.

Quality performance is usually measured and publicly reported at the hospital level. Physicians participate in hospital quality efforts on peer-review and credentialing committees. Some hospitals have well-organized efforts for continuous quality improvement. A published analysis of what works at the hospital level identified four factors that are critical to the success of a local quality -improvement effort: 1) high-level administrative support, 2) physician buy-in, 3) an explicit statement of the shared goals, and 4) a mechanism for measurement and feedback.[9] Other research has identified methods, such as simple checklists and "bundles" of care, that can improve quality.[10] Another simple method is the "time out," a practice used in operating and procedure rooms that forces operators to stop and recite a checklist of critical items before beginning a procedure.[11]

In our hospital, we developed a mechanism to give rapid feedback of reliable data on procedural performance to interventional cardiologists and cardiac surgeons. The reform has created an almost automatic mechanism to improve procedural quality. We developed a multidisciplinary committee to track procedural data using the ACC's National Cardiovascular Data Registry and the registry developed by the Society of Thoracic Surgeons. Our committee monitors program-wide performance and works to redesign systems if problems are identified.[12]

Figure 8.6 Door to balloon times at one hospital from January 2006 to September 2007 showing a steady improvement.

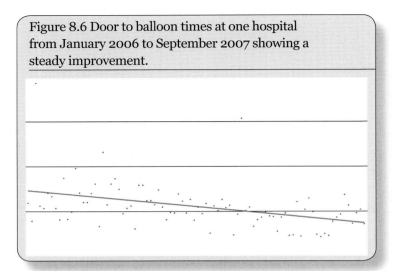

Figure 8.7 Example of a control chart, showing upper and lower control limits and the distribution of measurements over time.

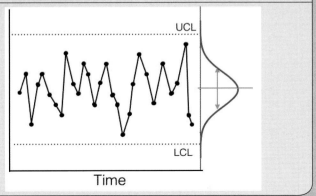

Figure 8.6 shows the door-to-balloon times from one of our hospitals for two years. This figure is an example of a control chart, a method of displaying system performance over time. Figure 8.7 shows the format of a standard control chart, with an upper and a lower control limit. Quality engineers Walter Shewhart and W. Edwards Deming used control charts to show variation in performance. They distinguished "chance causes" from "assignable causes" of variation.[13] System deficiencies result in assignable cause variation. Detecting this type of variation should lead to system redesign. Both Shewhart and Deming recognized that overreacting to chance causes, or the "noise" in measurement, leads to wasted quality-improvement efforts and may lower staff morale and foster an atmosphere of fear. Using data properly is key to successful local quality improvement.

In 2007, I had the privilege of working with the American College of Cardiology to help organize a nationwide quality-improvement initiative called D2B: An Alliance for Quality. This initiative sought to improve door-to-balloon times for patients admitted with ST-segment elevation myocardial infarction.[14] Before our initiative, outcomes research showed that only about 45% of STEMI patients were treated within a door-to-balloon time of <90 minutes, as recommended by clinical guidelines. Further study showed that some hospitals achieved extraordinary success, and this research identified several factors associated with consistently better door-to-balloon times.[15] Our quality-improvement initiative created a mechanism to share these best practices. We encouraged all participating hospitals to implement the successful strategies used by the high-performing hospitals. We enrolled more than 1000 hospitals nationwide.

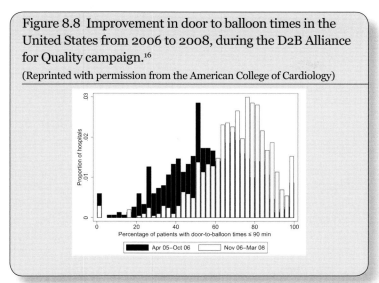

Figure 8.8 Improvement in door to balloon times in the United States from 2006 to 2008, during the D2B Alliance for Quality campaign.[16]
(Reprinted with permission from the American College of Cardiology)

From before the initiative in 2006 to after the initiative in 2008, the proportion of hospitals achieving improved door-to-balloon times increased substantially, as shown in Figure 8.8.[16] Further analysis showed that the door-to-balloon times in the U.S. improved considerably from 2005 to 2010 (Figure 8.9). The percentage of patients with a door-to-balloon time of <90 minutes rose from 45% in 2005 to more than 90% in 2010.[17] Other efforts, such as public reporting, and pay for performance may have had an effect, but the data clearly documented an enormous improvement during the timeframe of the D2B initiative, in a measure that had previously been resistant to improvement.

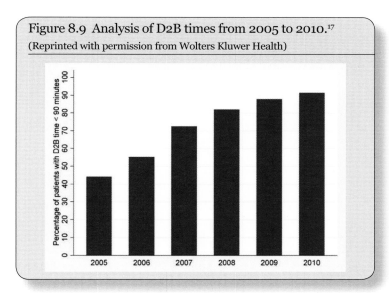

Figure 8.9 Analysis of D2B times from 2005 to 2010.[17]
(Reprinted with permission from Wolters Kluwer Health)

The D2B: Alliance for Quality initiative showed that focused efforts can improve the quality of care. The initiative encouraged hospitals to redesign their processes and to develop a mechanism for measuring and obtaining feedback about their door-to-balloon times. The initiative encouraged hospitals to replicate

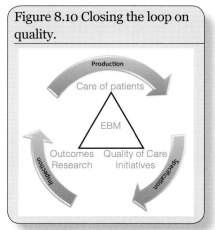

Figure 8.10 Closing the loop on quality.

what Walter Shewhart taught us in 1939: We can improve quality by "closing the loop." To close the loop, we define quality, and we create a means of production and inspection to ensure quality (Figure 8.10).

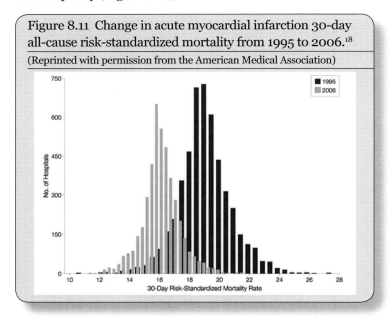

Figure 8.11 Change in acute myocardial infarction 30-day all-cause risk-standardized mortality from 1995 to 2006.[18]
(Reprinted with permission from the American Medical Association)

Substantial evidence shows that quality-improvement efforts are paying off. The 30-day risk standardized mortality for acute myocardial infarction in the U.S. has dropped by a relative 30% from 1995 to 2006 (Figure 8.11).[18] The distribution of the data in Figure 8.11 shows that we are making quality better and more reliable.

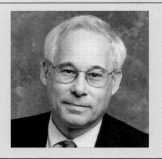

The Triple Aim

Donald Berwick, M.D.

1. Better care for individuals

2. Better care for populations

3. Reducing per-capita costs

Where do we go from here? Don Berwick has called for a "triple aim": 1) better care for individuals, 2) better care for populations, and 3) reducing per-capita costs of healthcare.[19] Achieving this aim will require a shift in our thinking. As physicians, we focus on individual patients, on the problem at hand. The triple aim forces us to think beyond each patient, each opportunity, and each procedure. Traditionally, we have focused on clinical care rather than the cost of care. Disregarding the cost of care is no longer possible. Dr. Berwick has challenged us to go beyond thinking about individual patients to thinking about a larger community of patients. Accountable care organizations and novel payment models may give us an incentive to start thinking along those lines.

References:

1. Committee on Quality of Health Care in America IOM. To err is human: Building a safer health system. Washington, DC: National Academy Press; 2000.

2. Committee on Quality of Health Care in America IOM. Crossing the quality chasm: A new health system for the 21st century. Washington, D.C.: National Academy Press; 2001.

3. Donabedian A. The quality of care. How can it be assessed? JAMA. 1988; 260:1743-1748

4. Tricoci P, Allen JM, Kramer JM, Califf RM, Smith SC, Jr. Scientific evidence underlying the ACC/AHA clinical practice guidelines. JAMA. 2009; 301:831-841

5. Patel MR, Spertus JA, Brindis RG, Hendel RC, Douglas PS, Peterson ED, Wolk MJ, Allen JM, Raskin IE, American College of Cardiology F. ACCF proposed method for evaluating the appropriateness of cardiovascular imaging. JACC. 2005; 46:1606-1613

6. Berwick DM, Godfrey AB, Roessner J. Curing health care: New strategies for quality improvement. San Fransisco, CA: Jossey-Bass Publishers; 1991.

7. Shewhart W. Statistical method from the viewpoint of quality control. Mineola, NY: Dover Pubilications; 1986 (Originally 1939).

8. Reason J. Human error. New York: Cambridge University Press; 1990.

9. Bradley EH, Holmboe ES, Mattera JA, Roumanis SA, Radford MJ, Krumholz HM. A qualitative study of increasing beta-blocker use after myocardial infarction: Why do some hospitals succeed? JAMA. 2001; 285:2604-2611

10. Pronovost P, Needham D, Berenholtz S, Sinopoli D, Chu H, Cosgrove S, Sexton B, Hyzy R, Welsh R, Roth G, Bander J, Kepros J, Goeschel C. An intervention to decrease catheter-related bloodstream infections in the ICU. N Eng J Med. 2006; 355:2725-2732

11. Gawande A. The checklist manifesto: How to get things right. New York: Metropolitan Books; 2010.

12. Brush JE, Jr., Balakrishnan SA, Brough J, Hartman C, Hines G, Liverman DP, Parker JP, Rich J, Tindall N. Implementation of a continuous quality improvement program for percutaneous coronary intervention and cardiac surgery at a large community hospital. American Heart Journal. 2006; 152:379-385

13. Deming WE. Out of the crisis. Cambridge, Mass.: Massachusetts Institute of Technology, Center for Advanced Engineering Study; 1986.

14. Krumholz HM, Bradley EH, Nallamothu BK, Ting HH, Batchelor WB, Kline-Rogers E, Stern AF, Byrd JR, Brush JE, Jr. A campaign to improve the timeliness of primary percutaneous coronary intervention: Door-to-balloon: An alliance for quality. JACC. Cardiovascular interventions. 2008; 1:97-104

15. Bradley EH, Herrin J, Wang Y, Barton BA, Webster TR, Mattera JA, Roumanis SA, Curtis JP, Nallamothu BK, Magid DJ, McNamara RL, Parkosewich J, Loeb JM, Krumholz HM. Strategies for reducing the door-to-balloon time in acute myocardial infarction. N Engl J Med. 2006; 355:2308-2320

16. Bradley EH, Nallamothu BK, Herrin J, Ting HH, Stern AF, Nembhard IM, Yuan CT, Green JC, Kline-Rogers E, Wang Y, Curtis JP, Webster TR, Masoudi FA, Fonarow GC, Brush JE, Jr., Krumholz HM. National efforts to improve door-to-balloon time results from the door-to-balloon alliance. JACC. 2009; 54:2423-2429

17. Krumholz HM, Herrin J, Miller LE, Drye EE, Ling SM, Han LF, Rapp MT, Bradley EH, Nallamothu BK, Nsa W, Bratzler DW, Curtis JP. Improvements in door-to-balloon time in the United States, 2005 to 2010. Circulation. 2011; 124:1038-1045

18. Krumholz HM, Wang Y, Chen J, Drye EE, Spertus JA, Ross JS, Curtis JP, Nallamothu BK, Lichtman JH, Havranek EP, Masoudi FA, Radford MJ, Han LF, Rapp MT, Straube BM, Normand SL. Reduction in acute myocardial infarction mortality in the united states: Risk-standardized mortality rates from 1995-2006. JAMA 2009; 302:767-773

19. Berwick DM, Nolan TW, Whittington J. The triple aim: Care, health, and cost. Health Affairs. 2008; 27:759-769

Chapter 9

Common Fallacies

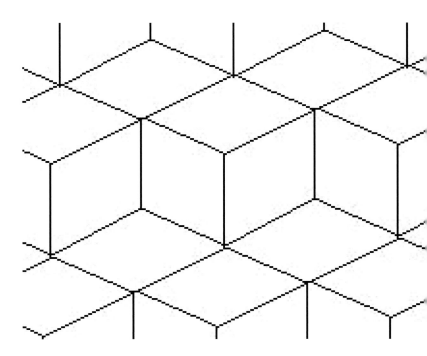

We often see what we want to see and believe what we want to believe. Look at the figure to the right. Are the boxes coming out of the page or going into the page? Now look at the picture on the following page (Figure 9.1). If you focus your gaze at the little nose on the left, the picture appears to be a young woman looking away. Focus on the large chin at the bottom, and the picture seems like an old woman looking toward you. You can make yourself see two different images. The same phenomenon applies to our thinking. We sometimes make ourselves believe what we want to believe. We can fool ourselves.

Visual illusions like Figure 9.1 are a good metaphor for mental illusions. Mental illusions can deceive us and lead us to conclusions that are fallacies — ones that defy the rules of logic and probability.

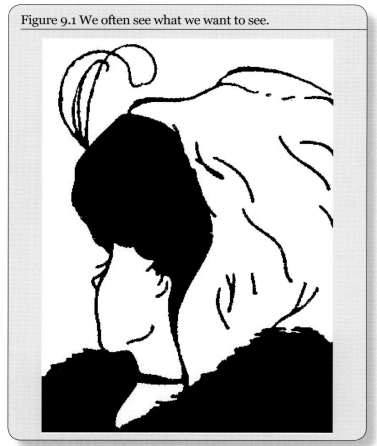

Figure 9.1 We often see what we want to see.

Some fallacies affect people in all occupations; some specifically affect doctors. Psychologists describe three types of fallacies: those that cause us to jump to conclusions, those that bias our judgments, and those that distort our probability estimates (Sidebar 9.1).[1] Psychologists say that we are particularly prone to hasty judgments, bias, and flawed probability estimates when we have incomplete information and when a decision is rushed. Incomplete information and rushed decisions are the norm in everyday medical practice, thereby leading practitioners to commit fallacies.

Hasty Judgments and System 1 Thinking

Bad judgment is often related to the malfunctioning of System 1 thinking, which was discussed in Chapter 2. Daniel Kahneman's *Thinking, Fast and Slow* is an excellent review of the fallibilities of System 1 thinking.[1]

System 1 thinking is intuitive; System 2 thinking is analytical. It seems logical that System 2 thinking should predominate in clinical medicine. However, the uncertainty that is an irreducible part of everyday clinical medicine makes it impossible to employ only System 2 thinking. We need System 1 thinking to interpolate, extrapolate, and make associations when crucial information is missing. System 1 comes up with creative solutions to unfamiliar problems; it gets us started when the problem at hand is unstructured.

System 1 thinking can also incorporate emotion and values into our judgments. Our patients, their families, and the public don't want us to reduce medical decision making merely to cold calculations and the strictly analytical approach of System 2 thinking. They want us to make value judgments, to add empathy. They want us to adjust the calculations when the circumstances demand special consideration. They want us to put the numbers in context.

Patients appreciate some aspects of System 1 thinking, but they also don't like mistakes. We are at our best when we monitor System 1 thinking and check our work with System 2 thinking. Good decision making requires that we reconcile our System 1 impulses with our System 2 calculations. We do that through an executive function called meta-cognition, or paying attention to how we think.

Kahneman describes System 1 thinking as an associative machine —a network whose nodes are ideas. System 1 pulls together many ideas, rapidly and sometimes unconsciously. Unfortunately, System 1 makes decisions based on what it sees and nothing more. It is not aware of alternatives and doesn't seek them out. Thus, System 1 can be a bit gullible and suggestible, often exaggerating the likelihood of unlikely events or propositions. System 2, in contrast, is vigilant and even suspicious. System 2 thinking can offer a backup to System 1 thinking; however, System 2 can be distracted and is sometimes lazy. When we go through the process of making a diagnosis, System 1 thinking gets us to envision various diagnostic possibilities, and System 2 thinking helps us examine those possibilities and construct a differential diagnosis. System 2 thinking helps us avoid jumping to conclusions by deliberately

organizing and expanding our thinking, and this requires active effort.

An example might be the evaluation of a patient with shortness of breath. System 1 thinking helps us see associations with other symptoms and bring various diagnostic possibilities to mind: recent hip surgery and a swollen leg might make us think of a pulmonary embolus, a productive cough and fever might bring pneumonia to mind, and orthopnea might make us think of congestive heart failure. System 2 thinking then takes over by forcing us to ask clarifying questions, expand the diagnostic possibilities, and engage in the process of iterative hypothesis testing that will enable us to confirm or reject a diagnosis.

System 1 tries to create coherence. It can jump to conclusions based on limited evidence. It is subject to overconfidence, framing effects, priming effects, and other biases. System 1 tends to ease cognitive strain by substituting an easier question for a harder one. Often, our patients do just that. If you ask a patient a question that requires a quantitative answer (e.g., "How long have you had that symptom?" "How long did it last?"), he or she will often evade the question and provide an answer to an easier question. We can correct for this tendency by repeating or reframing the question for the patient. Sometimes a multiple-choice question can let the patient know the type of answer we are seeking: "Has the pain been bothering you for a week or a month? Did the pain last a minute, or an hour? How long?" For ourselves, we can correct this mistake by monitoring System 1 activity and forcing our thinking back on track.

Biased Judgments

Our thinking can be affected by priming, whereby unconscious thoughts influence our ideas, emotions, and actions. This can take many forms, such as stereotyping, overconfidence, risk aversion, or dread. Our emotions can have a halo affect, influencing our thinking in imperceptible ways.

Stereotyping, which affects everyone's thinking, is the subject of the Institute of Medicine's 2003 book *Unequal Treatment: Confronting Racial and Ethnic Disparities in Health Care.*[2] Figure 9.2 shows that racial disparities in medical care can stem from multiple factors, including access to care, patient preferences, bias, prejudice, as well as stereotyping. The IOM book defined stereotyping as "the process by which people use social categories (e.g., race, sex) in acquiring, processing, and recalling information about others." Stereotyping can have powerful unconscious effects, even among well-meaning and well-educated people who are not overtly biased. Stereotyping can also affect the behavior of patients, who may react to

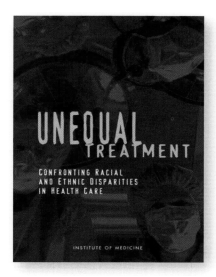

Figure 9.2 Figure from *Unequal Treatment* showing that differences in health care quality may be appropriate if due to patient preferences. Disparities in quality may be due to systems problems, or discrimination related to stereotyping.[2]

(Reprinted with permission from The National Academies Press)

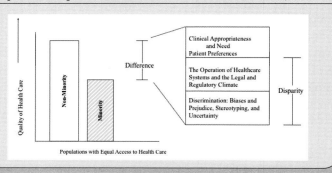

overt or subtle attitudes and the behaviors of their providers. Stereotyping can occur in the context of time pressure, resource constraints, and high cognitive demand.

Other forms of priming can affect our thinking in both positive and negative ways. Our medical school education imbued most of us with a sense of professionalism. We were primed with a sense of duty to the patient and a need to preserve the sanctity of the doctor-patient relationship. This professionalism can favorably influence our medical decisions. There is also a growing trend toward an entrepreneurial spirit in medicine. This may spur creativity and innovation, but it may also have adverse priming effects related to greed and conflict of interest. There are too many examples when doctors make treatment decisions based on greed, ignoring their duty to the welfare of their patients.

Medical malpractice concerns can have a priming effect on medical decision making. We have all heard vivid stories about colleagues who have been sued. To most doctors, the malpractice system seems capricious and unfair. The priming effect of malpractice fear can distort our thinking, resulting in defensive medicine. The fear of a malpractice suit is often disproportionate to the actual probability that a suit will be filed. The very prospect of a suit can prime decisions, leading to over-testing, over-interpreting test results, and over-treatment of patients.

Our thinking is also primed by financial incentives and rewards. Today, most of us practice in a fee-for-service world, which creates an incentive for thinking that more is better. An alternative payment model, prospective payment, also may have unintended effects on our thinking. Some suggest that prospective payment models could cause physicians to stint on care. Unfortunately, no payment model provides perfect incentives for promoting hard work and rational decisions.

Pay for performance, a "buzz phrase" in recent years, has as its goal paying for quality care rather than the quantity of services rendered. Questions remain about how well these payment models incentivize good thinking. Some believe that such models might cause people to think only about what is being rewarded, at the expense of other important aspects of patient care — much like "teaching to the test," when teachers narrow what they teach because their pay is tied to test scores.

Also, pay for performance will have little effect on our thinking if the rewards are insufficient or delayed. The hope of payment reform is to create incentives for doctors to choose diagnostic and therapeutic strategies that truly matter and create value for patients.[3]

Our perspective and frame of reference can also affect our decisions. Prospect theory, developed by Daniel Kahneman and Amos Tversky, explains how we weigh a decision depending on whether we surmise that it will lead to a potential gain or a potential loss. The prospect of a loss has more influence on decisions than does the prospect of an equal gain. Perhaps that explains why most physicians prefer to make an error of commission rather than omission.

Distorted Probability Estimates

We tend to overweight the probabilities of events or propositions at the extremes. The "possibility effect" makes us think that rare things are not only possible, but probable: "I think this patient probably has a pheochromocytoma." We also can have an illusion of certainty when we are way too certain about something that, objectively, is not certain at all: "I'm sure that this patient has an aortic dissection." The illusion of certainty can lead to arrogance. We all know an arrogant colleague who is sometimes wrong but is always certain. There is a big difference between self-confidence and arrogance. Having a little humility in medicine is an easy way to avoid the illusion of certainty and overconfidence. According to Gary Klein, a psychologist who has studied the intuition of experts, true experts know the limits of their knowledge.[4]

Kahneman and Tversky have described the availablity heuristic, whereby we give undue influence to events that are salient, recent, or easily remembered. For example, we may see a dramatic case of aortic dissection and then be more prone to make that diagnosis subsequently, even though the probability of the diagnosis is low.

Another fallacy described by Kahneman and Tversky is the representativeness heuristic. This fallacy places too much emphasis on resemblance to prior experiences, at the expense of a balanced, objective assessment of probability. For example, a patient may present with a classic appearance of pheochromocytoma, but the diagnosis would still be a bad bet because it is extremely rare. We have an adage in medicine: "When you hear hoofbeats, you should think horses, not zebras."

Anchoring and adjusting can lead to two types of fallacies (previously discussed in Chapter 3). One, simply called anchoring, is when we become attached to an initial impression and fail to change our thinking despite compelling new information. The second fallacy, base-rate neglect, leads us to forget to make an initial estimate of a prior probability and to base our judgment solely on the strength of new information. For example, a clinician may take the results of a stress test at face value, even though the patient has a very low prior probability of coronary artery disease.

Sidebar 9.1 Some Common Fallacies

Hasty Judgments:

- System 1 sees what it sees and nothing more.
- System 1 is often gullible.
- System 1 can mistakenly attribute cause and effect. *Post hoc, ergo propter hoc.*

Biased Judgments:

- Priming, stereotyping, halo effect of our emotions.
- Overconfidence, arrogance, ego bias, illusion of control.
- Risk aversion, defensive medicine, dread, regret.
- Prospect of losing has more impact on decisions than the prospect of an equal gain.
- Value-driven bias, wishful thinking, greed.
- Hindsight bias-memory conforms to the desired story.
- Confirmation bias-selective use of the facts.

Distorted Probability Estimates:

- Overweigh probability at the extremes
- Illusion of certainty
- Availability-undue influence of salient or recent events.
- Representativeness-too much emphasis on resemblance.
- Anchoring, base-rate neglect, denominator neglect.
- Gambler's fallacy, regression to the mean.

Many other fallacies have been described. The gambler's fallacy is a faulty prediction when we incorrectly see an interaction between events that are really independent. For example, we may be asked to interpret a series of tests. If by chance, many tests in a row are positive, we could think, "they cannot all be positive." This thinking could create bias and lead us to interpret the next test as negative, rather than interpreting each test independently and without bias. Another fallacy, regression to the mean, involves ascribing significance to a change in a result when the change is actually due to chance, causing the measurement to return to a point of central tendency. This fallacy could cause us to misinterpret trends in performance. For example, in being asked to measure our performance on patient satisfaction, we may find that the measure fell from one timeframe to the next. This shift might be attributable merely to natural variability, which is likely to regress to the mean, but the drop could instead be misinterpreted as a downward trend in performance.

Chapter 2 discussed the "Harvard Medical School problem," whereby doctors became confused and incorrectly answered a seemingly simple problem. When given the false-positive rate of a test and asked to identify the meaning of a positive result, the doctors tried to calculate predictive value from sensitivity and specificity, missing the fact that the parameters have different denominators. Using percentages contributed to the problem, because percentages can cause us to forget what the denominator represents. Using natural frequencies to define rates can help us avoid this so-called "denominator neglect." (Revisit chapter 2 for the numerical specifics.)

Fallacies of "Medical Heuristics"

Chapter 3 mentioned several habits or "medical heuristics" that are traditionally taught to each generation of medical trainees. These heuristics can help us organize and process cues, leading to rapid decisions. They can also be harmful when used improperly.

Early hypothesis generation helps us converge on a diagnosis by leading us to ask more-specific questions. It narrows the cognitive problem space, making the problem-solving exercise more efficient. By considering several leading possible diagnoses early in the patient interview, we can start a line of questioning that helps us home in on the diagnosis.

However, early hypothesis generation can also lead to mistakes. We need to remember that an early hypothesis is just that: a hypothesis, and not a conclusion. Jumping to conclusions, or "hasty generalization," is a well-known fallacy. Early hypothesis generation can sometimes lead to premature closure of the fact-finding exercise — specifically, to "diagnosis momentum," whereby we get stuck on one hypothesis and don't adequately consider alternatives. Use of a differential diagnosis can help us avoid jumping to a hasty conclusion by broadening our list of possibilities. Use of the differential diagnosis requires System 2 thinking. Avoiding hasty generalization requires active thinking and meta-cognition.

Expert physicians use a clinical narrative to articulate a coherent summary of a complex clinical case. Although the narrative can be helpful, it can also lead to problems. Nassem Taleb describes the narrative fallacy in his book *The Black Swan*.[5] According to Taleb, the narrative can be abused and turned into a misleading story. Trial lawyers know this well. They use narratives to persuade juries to agree with their point of view. Each lawyer makes use of confirmation bias to tell a completely different narrative, based roughly on the same set of facts. So facts can be manipulated to fit a desired narrative. We could fall into this trap when we evaluate patients with chest pain. Historical details can be emphasized or downplayed to make the history more consistent with musculoskeletal injury, pleurisy, angina, or whatever diagnosis we want.

Along with the narrative fallacy and confirmation bias, hindsight bias can cause our memory to conform to a desired story. Chapter 5 mentioned a fallacy called post hoc, ergo propter hoc, which translates "after this, therefore because of this." This fallacy describes how we can sometimes ascribe causality to events that occurred merely by coincidence.

Our System 1 thinking likes a good story and can sometimes draw the wrong meaning from the story. To avoid that problem, we need to follow the facts to the truth rather than creating a narrative that conforms to a preconceived story. A narrative is essential for organizing cues to make a problem recognizable, but use of the narrative can backfire if we are blind to its potential pitfalls.

Pat Croskerry has cataloged many common medical fallacies (see Sidebar 9.2),[6] calling them "cognitive dispositions to respond." He encourages greater awareness of these

---

Sidebar 9.2 Crokskerry's catalogue of biases and fallacies that lead to medical error.[6]

Aggregate bias	Sutton's slip
Anchoring	Sunk costs
Ascertainment bias	Triage cueing
Availability	Unpacking principle
Base-rate neglect	Vertical line failure
Commission bias	Visceral bias
Confirmation bias	Yin-Yang out
Diagnosis momentum	
Feedback sanction	
Framing effect	
Fundamental attribution error	
Gambler's fallacy	
Gender bias	
Hindsight bias	
Multiple alternatives bias	
Omission bias	
Order effects	
Outcome bias	
Overconfidence bias	
Playing the odds: (also known as frequency gambling)	
Posterior probability error	
Premature closure	
Psych-out error	
Representativeness restraint	
Search satisfying	

tendencies, greater use of metacognition, and the use of "cognitive forcing strategies." A cognitive forcing strategy is a method to consciously counteract a specific bias or fallacy. A mental strategy that can facilitate better thinking is to actively ask yourself, "Am I framing this right? Am I biased? Might I be stereotyping?" Jerry Kassirer also described many of these fallacies in his excellent book on medical reasoning.[7] With greater awareness of these fallacies, we can avoid predictable traps.

Another safeguard against biased thinking is consistent feedback and follow-up. We can calibrate our judgments by reviewing their accuracy through diligent follow-up and objective assessment. Case-by-case follow-up can help us gauge our ability to make a clinical diagnosis: "Did that patient pan out to have a pulmonary embolus after all?" Follow-up on individual cases is important, but the habit of measurement and feedback of aggregated performance is even better for calibrating our judgment: "What were the outcomes for the last 20 patients whom I referred for coronary artery bypass surgery?" By assessing our performance over time, with a sufficient sample size, we can objectively assess our performance and recalibrate when necessary.

Errors Due to the Task Environment

Many mental mistakes arise from the task environment in which we work. We labor under time pressures when we treat medical emergencies or when we are over-scheduled. Our medical decisions are almost always rushed. In addition, we are frequently distracted by beepers, cellphones, and interruptions from coworkers who demand our immediate attention. Like a driver who is texting, we multitask and make rapid decisions while being bombarded by distractions.

We are also often fatigued, a problem of our own creation because of tight call schedules and long working hours. Studies have shown that fatigued doctors resemble drunken drivers in how their decision-making capacity is impaired.[8]

Charles Perrow describes how working conditions and high-risk tasks can conspire to cause catastrophes.[9] In his book *Normal Accidents*, he classifies interactions that occur in a work environment as either linear or complex, and as either loosely or tightly coupled. A hospital is a complex system. The tasks are loosely coupled in some areas and tightly coupled in others. For example, the hospital shipping department is complex and loosely coupled, whereas the pharmacy is more linear and tightly coupled. Problems arise in areas that are complex and tightly coupled. The emergency room, the operating room, and the cardiac catheterization lab can become complex and tightly coupled during emergencies. These environments are like the flight deck of an aircraft carrier, where things can go bad quickly, but standard operating procedures, checklists, timeouts, and other routines can focus thinking, improve performance, and prevent adverse outcomes.[10,11]

Good environments lead to good thinking, which leads to good decisions and good outcomes. Paying attention to the environmental challenges of the workplace and challenges related to scheduling, overwork, and distractions can improve the quality of our decisions and reduce errors.

Most mistakes in judgment stem from jumping to conclusions, making biased decisions, or using distorted estimates of probability. Many of these mistakes can be avoided if we monitor our thinking.

References:

1. Kahneman D. Thinking, fast and slow. New York: Farrar, Straus and Giroux; 2011.

2. Smedley BD, Stith AY, Nelson AR, Institute of Medicine (U.S.). Committee on understanding and eliminating racial and ethnic disparities in health care. Unequal treatment: Confronting racial and ethnic disparities in health care. Washington, D.C.: National Academy Press; 2003.

3. De Brantes F, Conte B. The incentive cure: The real relief for health care. Amazon Kindle Edition; 2013.

4. Klein, Gary. The power of intuition. New York: Random House; 2003.

5. Taleb N. The black swan: The impact of the highly improbable. New York: Random House; 2007.

6. Croskerry P. Cognitive forcing strategies in clinical decision making. Ann Emerg Med. 2003; 41:110-120

7. Kassirer JP, Wong JB, Kopelman RI. Learning clinical reasoning. Baltimore, MD: Lippincott Williams & Wilkins Health; 2010.

8. Samkoff JS, Jacques CH. A review of studies concerning effects of sleep deprivation and fatigue on residents' performance. Acad Med 1991; 66:687-693

9. Perrow C. Normal accidents : Living with high-risk technologies. Princeton, N.J.: Princeton University Press; 1999.

10. Pronovost P, Needham D, Berenholtz S, Sinopoli D, Chu H, Cosgrove S, Sexton B, Hyzy R, Welsh R, Roth G, Bander J, Kepros J, Goeschel C. An intervention to decrease catheter-related bloodstream infections in the ICU. The New England Journal of Medicine. 2006; 355:2725-2732

11. Gawande A. The checklist manifesto: How to get things right. New York: Metropolitan Books; 2010.

Chapter 10

Putting This Book Into Practice

"Principles for the development of a complete mind: Study the science of art. Study the art of science."

- Leonardo da Vinci

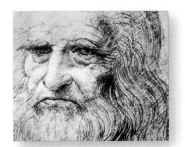

Leonardo da Vinci (1452-1519)

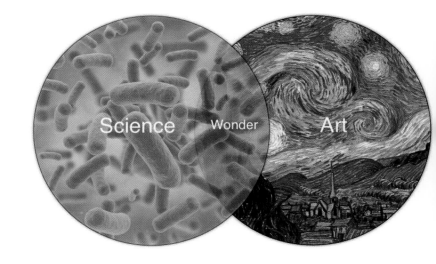

I started educating myself about medical reasoning because I wanted to improve the quality of clinical care. I initially assumed that most medical mistakes stem from poor judgment and that simply educating people about fundamental axioms of medical practice would be the key to improving quality. I learned, though, that the problem isn't so simple.

Sure, medicine has its axioms, rules, algorithms, dictums, aphorisms, values, habits, and decision aids. We have Occam's razor (multiple clinical findings are most likely attributable to a single condition), the zebra rule (common things are common, just as the sound of hoof beats is more likely to come from horse than a zebra), and Sutton's Law (go directly to the source, like Willie Sutton, who said that he robbed banks because that's where the money was). We have guiding values, such as a commitment to thoroughness, direct observation, science, and patient-centeredness. We have habits that become default behaviors and routines. We have computerized decision support, mnemonics, and reminder systems to guide our thinking.

Those thinking-support tools are helpful but not sufficient for making most medical decisions. Almost all everyday decisions in clinical medicine demand the use of intuition. As Herbert Simon said, "Intuition is nothing more and nothing less than recognition." Intuition helps us make associations and develop creative solutions, but it can also lead to mistakes. In short, intuition is both a strength and a weakness.

To improve the quality of care, we must therefore deepen our understanding of how we use intuition and how we can calibrate it with science and objective data. The purpose of this book is to help the reader achieve those decision-making goals at the bedside of each patient.

No one should assume that using intuition in medicine means "winging it." It involves drawing on what psychologists call "expert intuition." According to Kahneman and Klein, two conditions are necessary for developing expert intuition: "First, the environment must provide adequately valid cues to the nature of the situation. Second, people must have the opportunity to learn the relevant cues."[1] Likelihood ratios, numbers needed to treat, and Bayes factors are ways that we can simplify and quantify the validity of the relevant cues and incorporate the objective science of medicine into our practice routines.

In their work on expert intuition, Chase and Simon found that if you show a chess board to a chess master for about 5 seconds, he will remember where most of the pieces are (unlike a novice, who recalls much less).[2] Experts are good at creating mental representations in their working memory and, with the benefit of experience, refining those representations and learning how to access them more quickly. Gary Klein has studied firefighter captains, field commanders, seasoned ICU nurses, and other experts to determine how recognition leads to good decisions in uncertain, rapidly changing, high-stakes situations.[3] He uses the term "recognition primed decision making" to describe how experts employ tacit knowledge and intuition to quickly size up a situation.

Norman and colleagues say that doctors develop expertise by acquiring both formal knowledge and experiential knowledge.[4] They learn the "what" and the "how." Experiential knowledge teaches the expert to, in Norman's words, "synthesize the details into a brief but coherent problem formulation, ignoring extraneous details." In short, experts know what they are looking at because they know what to look for.

Herbert Simon taught us that we tackle structured decisions and unstructured problems differently. For structured decisions, we use inductive reasoning and probability. Conditional probability and Bayes' Rule give us a way to think about structured decisions. For many structured decisions, we intuitively estimate the probabilities using the anchoring and adjusting heuristic. For unstructured problems, we rely on a variety of heuristics that enable us to link together various cues in a useful structure. Many of the routines that are traditionally taught in medical training are like heuristics. They are processes that help us organize complex information and give shape to an unstructured problem.

Our intuition can be fooled, though, and cognitive psychologists identify three types of fallacies: those that cause us to jump to conclusions, those that bias our judgments, and those that distort our probability estimates. They say that we are particularly prone to these errors when we have incomplete information and when a decision is rushed, as is the norm in everyday practice. We can avoid errors by developing good habits, by checking our work using metacognition, and by maintaining good work environments that foster clear thinking, sound decisions, and better outcomes.

Effective use of intuition requires practice, of course. The psychologist Anders Ericsson has analyzed how "practice makes perfect" by studying musicians, athletes, and high achievers in other domains.[5] Repetitive practice brings people to proficiency, but achieving expert performance requires goal-oriented and focused deliberate practice.[6,7] It demands motivation and concentration, uses critical self-evaluation, and is mindful of every opportunity for learning. With deliberate practice, experts internalize their skills to the point of near-automation. Sidebar 10.1 lists goals for learning and practicing some of the ideas in this book in a deliberate fashion.

In the preface, I noted that medical education focuses primarily on teaching the "what" rather than the "how." Toward that end, I believe that teaching the "how" should be very visual and interactive. Words on a page or in a lecture often have little effect on System 1 thinking. Two-dimensional visual explanations, like those in this book, are more effective. Three-dimensional, real-life examples and experiences have the greatest influence.[8] When medical students and residents engage in active problem solving using real-life examples, they have the opportunity to think more critically about the structure of their decisions.

Simon and others estimate that it takes about 10,000 hours for an expert to learn the "how." If you work 68 hours per week, 49 weeks per year, for 3 years, you will log 9,996 hours. The duration of residency and fellowship training barely gives trainees enough time to become experts. I hope that this book will give trainees a better understanding of the skills they aim to acquire, so that they can develop expert intuition earlier, more efficiently, and more reliably.

Unfortunately, making optimal medical decisions is hard. We often face stress and fatigue, are constrained by time, and lack sufficient data. We also tolerate constant uncertainty, which we tame through the use of reasoning. Some situations allow us to just follow simple rules, but most clinical situations require complex integration of scientific principles with our intuition to generate commonsense, practical solutions.

Medical reasoning is baffling to people outside medicine and, often, to medical practitioners themselves. The practice of medicine is an art, but close examination reveals more order and regularity than is initially apparent. There is a science to the art of medicine. When we integrate scientific precision and elegantly simple intuition with each patient's personal preferences and values, we can offer high-quality medical care that is a scientifically rigorous work of art.

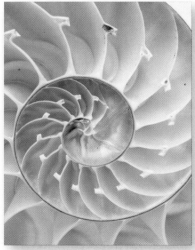

Close inspection of the art of medicine reveals more order and regularity than is initially apparent.

References:

1. Kahneman D, Klein G. Conditions for intuitive expertise: A failure to disagree. American Psychologist 64(6); 515-526: 2009.

2. Chase WG, Simon HA. The mind's eye in chess. In W.G.Chase (Ed.), Visual information processing. New York: Academic Press; 1973.

3. Klein G. The power of intuition. New York: Random House; 2003.

4. Norman G, Eva K, Brooks L, Hamstra S. Expertise in Medicine and Surgery. In Ericsson KA, et al. The Cambridge handbook of expertise and expert performance. Cambridge; New York: Cambridge University Press; 2006.

5. Ericsson KA. Deliberate practice and acquisition and maintenance of expert performance in medicine and related domains. Academic Medicine 79(10);S70-S81:2004.

6. Ericsson KA. The influence of experience and deliberate practice on the development of superior expert performance. In Ericsson KA. The Cambridge handbook of expertise and expert performance. Cambridge; New York: Cambridge University Press; 2006.

7. Hogarth RM. Educating intuition. Chicago: University of Chicago Press. 2001.

8. Kassirer JP. Teaching clinical reasoning: Case-based and coached. Academic Medicine 2010; 85(7):1118-1124

Appendices

Appendix 1

More on Probability Curves

Many points in this book are illustrated using normal or "bell-shaped" probability curves. The formula for the normal curve was derived by the German mathematician, C. F. Gauss.[1] The curve is also called a Gaussian curve or Gaussian distribution. The formula for the curve is shown below.

$$f(x) = \frac{1}{\sqrt{2\pi\sigma^2}} e^{-\frac{(x-\mu)^2}{2\sigma^2}}$$

The formula for the normal curve looks pretty daunting to a non-mathematician like me, but if we break it down, we can discover a couple of interesting things about the formula.

First, the function that defines the shape of the normal curve is determined by two parameters: the mean (μ) and the standard deviation (σ) of a sample.

Second, the exponent of e is negative. Therefore, the e-term (circled in red) is a fraction. The e-term maximizes to 1 when the exponent of e is 0. The exponent of e is 0 when

the x-coordinate equals the mean of a sample (when $x=\mu$). Therefore, the height of the curve [f(x) or the y-coordinate] is maximized in the middle of the curve at the point where $x=\mu$.

Third, the shape of the curve is determined by the standard deviation of a sample. Since the e-term equals 1 at $x=\mu$, the height of the curve at $x=\mu$ is determined by the remaining part of the function: $1/\sqrt{(2\pi\sigma^2)}$. The standard deviation (σ) is in the denominator of this function, so the height of the curve at $x=\mu$ is inversely proportional to the standard deviation. For any sample distribution, the maximum probability (the mode of the curve) increases as the standard deviation of the sample decreases. We can plug some numbers into the formula to demonstrate this: For a $\sigma=4$, the height of the curve is approximately 0.10. For a $\sigma=2$, the height of the curve is approximately 0.20. For $\sigma=1$, the height of the curve is approximately 0.40, as shown.

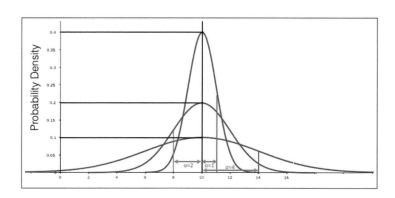

One standard deviation on either side of the mean defines an area under the curve or a cumulative probability of 0.68. Two standard deviations (actually 1.96) defines a cumulative probability of 0.95. Three standard deviations defines a cumulative probability of 0.99.

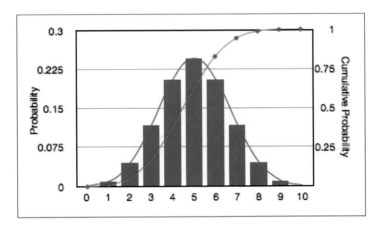

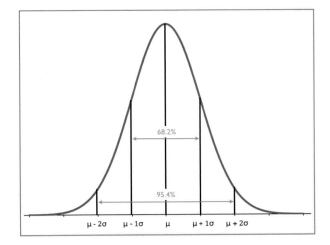

Most likely, 5 heads will turn up. Next most likely is either 4 heads or 6 heads, and so on. If we flip 100 coins repeatedly, we can create a binomial distribution that starts to look like a normal curve.

These curves describe probability over a range of possibilities where the x-axis is a continuous variable. Other variables that we discuss in this book are discrete variables. For example, many clinical trials report binary outcomes such as mortality. For a binary variable, we can create a binary distribution.

An example of a binary variable is a coin toss, where the outcome is either heads or tails. If we repeatedly flip 10 coins at a time and record the number of heads each time, we can create a binary distribution, shown below.

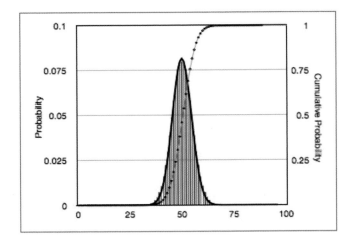

141

The shape of a normal curve and its location on the x-axis determines how a curve would overlap with another probability curve. Statistical principles and calculations are based on how normal curves overlap and interact. We will use normal curves in this book to explain diagnostic tests, likelihood ratios, and Bayes factors. Knowing some of the properties of normal curves will help us later when we use normal curves to understand these concepts.

Reference:

1. Hacking I. An introduction to probability and inductive logic. Cambridge, U.K.; New York; Cambridge University Press; 2001.

Appendix 2
More on Likelihood Ratios

The idea of likelihood was proposed by R.A.Fisher and discussed by Ian Hacking in his book, Logic of Statistical Inference.[1] Likelihood ratios give us a way to make an inference about a patient's test result based on the known operating characteristics of the test. The operating characteristics of the test, namely the sensitivity and specificity, are determined in a research setting. Research gives us the frequencies of positive and negative test results among patients known to have disease and among people known not to have disease. Researchers use these frequencies to calculate sensitivity and specificity of the test.

What can a single test result tell us about a unique case in practice, given the operating characteristics of a test? Likelihood ratios give us a way to know how a test result should shift our thinking about an individual patient.

To explain likelihood ratios, we can borrow the analogy that Daniel Bernoulli used in 1777 to explain variation. He used an example of an archer shooting arrows at a target. We will use Bernoulli's analogy and modify it to create an example that explains likelihood ratios.

Imagine an archer and two targets, a blue target and a red target, placed side-by-side. The targets overlap and are placed a certain distance apart (x). The archer shoots a series of blue arrows at the blue target and a series of red arrows at the red

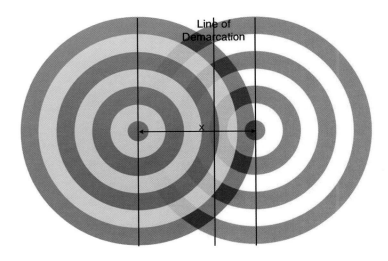

target. The archer is good, but not perfect, so there is some scatter of the arrows around each bull's eye.

After the archer shoots the series of blue and red arrows at the blue and red targets, we then measure the horizontal distances of the arrows from the two bull's eyes and we plot the distances using probability density curves, as shown below.

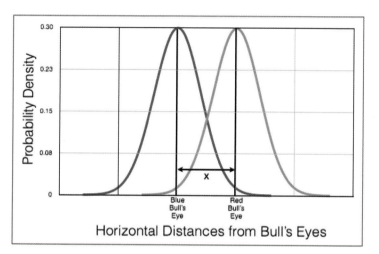

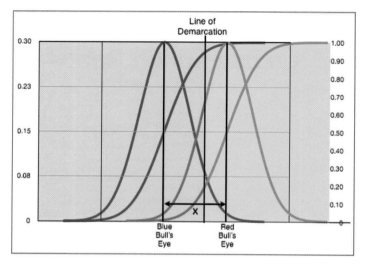

We then decide to draw a line between the two bull's eyes so that 95% of the blue arrows are to the left of the line and 80% of the red arrows are to the right of the line. This line of demarcation would separate the blue arrows from the red arrows with a sensitivity of 95% and a specificity of 80%. In other words, the area to the left of the line would capture the blue arrows with a 0.95 true positive rate and a 0.20 false positive rate. The line is shown on the targets above and on the probability density curves and the cumulative probability curves below.

Having established the setup, let's suppose that the archer now shoots another arrow, which is white. He shoots the white arrow at one of the targets, but doesn't reveal which one he aimed at. The white arrow lands to the left of the line. How certain are we that the archer was aiming at the blue target?

Based on our setup (the distance between the bull's eyes, where we placed our line of demarcation, and the observed frequencies of the blue and red arrows on either side of the line), we can make an inference about which target the white arrow was aimed at. The true positive rate of 0.95 supports the notion that the arrow was aimed at the blue target. The false positive rate of 0.2 supports the notion that the arrow was aimed at the red target. The support for the blue target is greater than the support for the red target by a ratio of 0.95 to 0.2, as shown on the cumulative probability curves below. This relative support is the likelihood ratio, which in this case is 0.95/0.2, or 4.75.

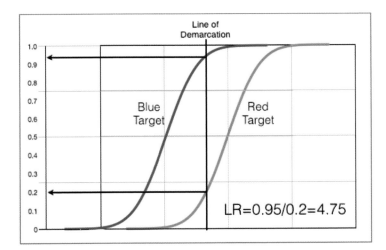

Our example is analogous to testing, where the blue target represents patients with disease and the blue arrows represent positive test results. The red target represents patients without disease and the red arrows represent negative test results. Blue arrows landing to the left of the line are true positives and red arrows landing to the left of the line are false positives. Red arrows landing to the right of the line are true negatives and blue arrows landing to the right of the line are false negatives. Depending on where we draw the line of demarcation, we can change the sensitivity and specificity to yield more or less true and false positive and negative test results. Once the operating characteristics of the test are determined, the sensitivity and specificity of the test can be used to easily calculate the positive and negative likelihood ratios for the test.

A likelihood ratio is dimensionless number. What does this number mean? A.W.F. Edwards wrote a book entitled *Likelihood*, in which he says that the meaning of likelihood becomes apparent with experience.[2] You have to live with likelihood ratios for a while to get a sense of their magnitude. As Hacking says, you may not be familiar with temperature measured in centigrade, but if you spend a summer in the south of France, you will learn what 30 degrees centigrade means. If you spend some time with likelihood ratios, you will learn what they mean.

To easily get a sense of the magnitude of likelihood ratios, we can create several examples where we multiply likelihood ratios by a prior odds of 1. A prior odds of 1 means that we are initially indifferent about some proposition (an odds of 1 equals a probability of 0.5). The prior odds times the likelihood ratio equals the posttest odds, which we can then convert to posttest probability (p=odds/1+odds). A likelihood ratio of 2 changes our prior odds of 1 to a posttest odds of 2, yielding a posttest probability of 2/3 or 0.67. A likelihood ratio of 5 yields a posttest probability of 5/6 or 0.83. A likelihood ratio of 10 yields a posttest probability of 10/11, or 0.91. Noodling around with likelihood ratios can give us an intuitive sense of their magnitude and how tests with different likelihood ratios should change our thinking about a unique case.

References:

1. Hacking I. Logic of Statistical Inference. Cambridge: Cambridge University Press, 1976.

2. Edwards AWE. Likelihood. Baltimore: The Johns Hopkins University Press, 1992.

Appendix 3

The Minimum Bayes Factor and Likelihood Ratios

As discussed in Chapter 4 and in Sidebar 4.1, likelihood ratios give us a way to make an inference about a test result, given the known operating characteristics of the test. Harold Jeffreys and I. J. Good and others proposed a way to use likelihood ratios to make an inference about a clinical trial.[1] When used for this purpose, the likelihood ratio is called the minimum Bayes factor. The Bayes factor gives us a way to make an inference about a clinical trial, given the trial's statistical parameters. The Bayes factor gives us a measure of the comparative support for the null hypothesis versus the support for the alternative hypothesis, as shown below.

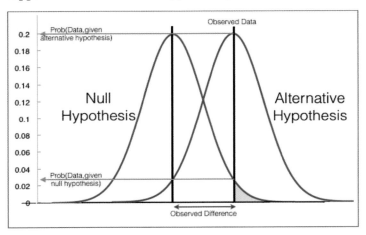

The formula for the Bayes factor is derived from the probability function of the null hypothesis divided by the probability function of the alternative hypothesis. The derivation is described in a review by Goodman.[1] The formula simplifies to the following formula:

Minimum Bayes factor $= e^{-z^2/2}$

Where $z = x/\sigma$, which is the observed difference, or treatment effect/the standard error of the observed data.

The Bayes factor can also be calculated from t-tests and chi-square tests.[1]

Bayes factors, like likelihood ratios, are handy because they are multipliers. The Bayes factor times the prior odds of the null hypothesis equals the posterior odds of the null hypothesis. As with likelihood ratios, with Bayes factors we have to convert prior probability into odds, and posterior odds back to probability.

In the example shown in the figure above, the Bayes factor is 0.03/0.2=0.15. A Bayes factor of 0.15 would change a prior probability of the null from 0.5 to a posterior probability of 0.13. It would change a prior probability of the null from 0.25 to 0.05.

References:

1. Goodman SN. Toward evidence-based medical statistics. 2: The Bayes Factor. Ann Intern Med 1999; 130(12):1005-1013

About the Author

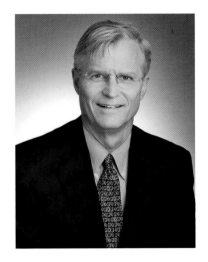

John E. Brush, Jr., M.D., FACC graduated from Hampden-Sydney College in 1976 and from the University of Virginia School of Medicine in 1980. He trained in Internal Medicine at the University of Vermont School of Medicine and in Cardiology at Yale University School of Medicine. From 1985 to 1988, he was a Senior Investigator and staff cardiologist with the Cardiology Branch of the National Institutes of Health in Bethesda, MD. From 1988 to 1992, he was on the faculty of Boston University School of Medicine. Since 1992, he has practiced cardiology in Norfolk, Virginia. He is a Professor of Medicine at Eastern Virginia Medical School and a cardiologist with Sentara Cardiology Specialists. He has served on a number of boards and committees of state and national organizations and including the Board of Trustees of the American College of Cardiology and the Cardiovascular Board of the American Board of Internal Medicine. Dr. Brush lives in Virginia Beach, VA with his wife, Gay Goldsmith, and two children, Evan and Anna.

Acknowledgements

Acknowledgments: A number of people reviewed previous drafts of this book and offered many thoughtful comments and suggestions. I would like to thank Robert Califf, MD, Daniel Mark, MD, Kevin Schulman, MD, and Kevin Weinfurt, Ph.D at Duke University; Harlan Krumholz, MD, SM, Vivek Kulkarni, Behnood Bikdeli, MD, and Ruijun Chen at Yale University; Robert Harrington, MD at Stanford University; Rick Nishimura, MD, and David Holmes, MD at the Mayo Clinic; Patrick O'Gara, MD at Harvard University, William Oetgen, MD, MBA at the American College of Cardiology, Allen Ciuffo, MD, John Parker, MD, Thad Waites, MD, David May, MD, Ph.D, and Elizabeth Thalhimer Smartt for their help. Also, I would like to thank Five Partners Foundation of New York, NY for their support, Amy Mendelson Cheeley and Wayne Dementi at Dementi Milestone Publishing, Jeffry Braun for the cover design, and Steve DeMaio for his expert editorial assistance.

When you write a book, you spend many hours working alone, away from family and friends. I would like to thank my wife, Gay Goldsmith, and my children, Evan and Anna, for tolerating my absence and for their love and support.